unDiet Yourself

unDiet Yourself

The No BS "Black Book"
Secrets To Get Fit Eating Fun Foods

Mitch Calvert

Disclaimer:

(1) Introduction This disclaimer governs the use of this book. [By using this book, you accept this disclaimer in full. / We will ask you to agree to this disclaimer before you can access the book.] No part of this book may be reproduced in any written, electronic, recording, or photocopying without written permission of the author. All trademarks are the exclusive property of mitchcalvert.com

(2) Credit This disclaimer was created using an SEQ Legal template.

(3) No advice The book contains information about men's dieting from the perspective of the author. The information is not advice, and should not be treated as such. You must not rely on the information in the book as an alternative to medical advice from an appropriately qualified professional. If you have any specific questions about any matter you should consult an appropriately qualified medical professional. If you think you may be suffering from any medical condition you should seek immediate medical attention. You should never delay seeking medical advice, disregard medical advice, or discontinue medical treatment because of information in this book

(4) No representations or warranties To the maximum extent permitted by applicable law and subject to section 6 below, we exclude all representations, warranties, undertakings and guarantees relating to the book. Without prejudice to the generality of the foregoing paragraph, we do not represent, warrant, undertake or guarantee: • that the information in the book is correct, accurate, complete or non-misleading; • that the use of the guidance in the book will lead to any particular outcome or result;

(5) Limitations and exclusions of liability The limitations and exclusions of liability set out in this section and elsewhere in this disclaimer: are subject to section 6 below; and govern all liabilities arising under the disclaimer or in relation to the book, including liabilities arising in contract, in tort (including negligence) and for breach of statutory duty. We will not be liable to you in respect of any losses arising out of any event or events beyond our reasonable control. We will not be liable to you in respect of any business losses, including without limitation loss of or damage to profits, income, revenue, use, production, anticipated savings, business, contracts, commercial opportunities or goodwill. We will not be liable to you in respect of any loss or corruption of any data, database or software. We will not be liable to you in respect of any special, indirect or consequential loss or damage.

(6) Exceptions Nothing in this disclaimer shall: limit or exclude our liability for death or personal injury resulting from negligence; limit or exclude our liability for fraud or fraudulent misrepresentation; limit any of our liabilities in any way that is not permitted under applicable law; or exclude any of our liabilities that may not be excluded under applicable law.

(7) Severability If a section of this disclaimer is determined by any court or other competent authority to be unlawful and/or unenforceable, the other sections of this disclaimer continue in effect. If any unlawful and/or unenforceable section would be lawful or enforceable if part of it were deleted, that part will be deemed to be deleted, and the rest of the section will continue in effect.

(8) Our details In this disclaimer, "we" means (and "us" and "our" refer to) Mitch Calvert (Manitoba, Canada) and team and or any future addresses, temporary or permanent."

TABLE OF CONTENTS

HE HAD A STEAK IN HIS POCKET

"Hey Mitch, have you tried this new Carnivore diet?"

The question came firing across the table as I dined with some members of a mentorship program I'm in.

We were at this fancy Italian restaurant known for their pasta (of course).

I said I had heard of it, and saw it was working wonders for some people, but didn't tell him how I really felt, knowing this gentleman—we'll call him Roger—was likely looking for validation.

Later, the server comes around and takes our orders. I ordered the bison meatball pasta based on her recommendation because my approach allows me to eat fun meals in moderation (more on that in a second).

She makes her way around the table and comes to Roger, the aforementioned gentleman who asked me about the Carnivore Diet earlier.

"Just water for me, thanks, I brought my own meal."

As soon as the server brings our food over, Roger here pulls out a tupperware container with some sort of ice cold steak, plain, with no side.

Now I'm curious, and ask him how he's managing to stick to it.

"Oh, the diet doesn't allow for carbs, so nothing on this menu works. It works fast for weight loss so I'm going to stick to my guns. I don't mind."

Wow, great, I thought, knowing the eventual outcome of this scenario was all too easy to predict.

Sure enough, a month later, I was curious and asked him at one of our Zoom meetings how it was going.

He replied "Oh, that carnivore thing? Yeah, I did lose some weight, but I crashed and burned last weekend and went on a carb bender. It was just too restrictive to stick to."

DING DING DING! Unfortunately, for most mere mortals like you and I, life doesn't fit the mold of fad diets.

You think you've found the silver bullet, but it doesn't last, because you're trying to plan your life around the diet, not the other way around.

Not to mention how awkward and challenging it is carrying around tupperware with a cold, dry steak at the ready.

Believe me, I've been there.

I was once frisked at a sports bar with a chicken breast in my pocket and vowed to never be that extreme again.

The key to a permanent body transformation is following a diet you enjoy and can stick to, while making small and sustainable sacrifices along the way.

That's what this book is about. It's the path to UnDiet Yourself. If you're looking for a quick fix fad that leaves you worse off than you started, return this book to Amazon, no hard feelings. In my opinion, the best diet is not a diet at all but a lifestyle you can stick to.

In fact, there's a simple Big Five framework that helped me lose 60 pounds in my 20s and has now done the same for thousands of Calvert Fitness members.

Dive into the book and you'll get a complete plan to tackle your weight, once and for all, without hang-ups, hurdles or hating your life.

Let's get to it...

MY GYM TEACHER CALLED ME FAT!

First, we start from the beginning, because that's how every story starts. I remember the moment I hit rock bottom.

It was a gym class in 2002 in my senior year at Shaftesbury High School. One of those hand-held body-fat measurement devices was making the rounds. I tried to avoid the test with an extended stay in the bathroom, but I was outed by a classmate.

The results told me everything I already knew: I was fat. The reading came up at 36 percent body fat — the worst score among the guys in the class.

People who try to lose weight often have a hard time committing to their goals. Accountability can go a long way in keeping you focused and on the right track.

That told me I needed to change, but I didn't know where to start.

I dabbled for several years after that, but you know where dabbling gets us: a big, fat nowhere.

So, what did I finally do to lose 53 pounds and keep it off going on 14 years now?

I stumbled upon a three-part formula that I now use with all my clients.

I remember the day it all changed. I was still living with my parents, a year removed from high school. I was working as a line cook at Grapes on Kenaston (RIP!) and had no real direction in my life, other than a legitimate addiction to video games and junk food.

I stared at myself in the mirror and got real that morning. I didn't say I needed to lose a couple pounds. No, I pointed at myself and said, "You're a fat SOB and this ends now."

I continued: "The mirror you see every day is going to tell you the truth every time, so why are you still lying to yourself? So you can convince yourself this is OK? It's not."

There was nothing healthy or fulfilling about the weight I carried. I knew it and you know it if you're in the same position or have been in the past.

There's no use sugar-coating it. But awareness is not enough. The commitment and action must follow suit.

HOW I LOST 60 POUNDS

You came here looking for the blueprint, and this book promises to share the tactics necessary to lose fat forever.

But it must start within. A combination of commitment, accountability and a potential loss is the formula to start.

What Is Loss Aversion? Loss aversion in behavioral economics refers to a phenomenon where a real or potential loss is perceived by individuals as psychologically or emotionally more severe than an equivalent gain.

In order to fully commit back in 2003, I told myself if I didn't lose 50 pounds, I'd quit playing video games for a year (a big deal to me at the time) and left a sticky note on my computer monitor to remind me.

I also enlisted my dad for accountability, who was more than happy to see me get off the computer. I didn't know it at the time, but this strategy is outlined in *The Blackmail Diet*, an obscure book by John Bear.

The author battles obesity and comes up with a plan: he signs a contract with a lawyer and puts US$5,000 in escrow. The contract states that if in a year's time the author doesn't lose 70 pounds, the lawyer must give all the money to the American Nazi Party.

As expected, a year later he had lost 70 pounds.

If you've struggled to lose weight and keep it off, it's probably because you treat it like that leaky sink in the downstairs bathroom. You'll get to it when the mood strikes.

You say things like:

"It's not the right time."

"I can't afford coaching right now."

"I'll start next Monday."

Most of the time, we don't fail to achieve our goals because of lack of knowledge and how-to, it's because we haven't associated the right level of motivation to the outcome.

What you need is something called a forcing function. A forcing function is any task, activity or event that forces you to take action and produce a result.

Let's start with a few real-world examples. In one instance, a client of mine was recently engaged and knew she wanted to look amazing in her wedding dress.

That gave her a forcing function to take action. She has the urgency and inspiration to commit to a plan now.

For another client, he was over 300 pounds and had tried countless times to lose the weight, with little success. It kept going the wrong direction.

But one day, his wife unexpectedly gave him some big news: she was pregnant. That was his forcing function. He knew things would be different this time because he wasn't taking no for an answer. He lost over 100 pounds and became the fit dad he envisioned becoming.

For others, it may be a divorce, health issue or some other arbitrary trigger that becomes the forcing function. Whatever it is, you need to find yours and pair it up with commitment and accountability.

With the combination of commitment, accountability and laser focus, I lost the weight within a year, and now, some 20 years later, I'm still doing my thing and coaching others to do the same within a similar framework. Your next diet attempt will be different if you start with this three-step process first.

WHY I DO WHAT I DO

I want to share the toughest moment in the history of Calvert Fitness with you today...

But, first, some quick background.

Picture a man on his couch... his name is Serge.

Obvious to anyone, he's carrying one too many pounds.

But look into his eyes and you see he has so much to offer deep inside.

Now picture a 6-year-old girl running into the room.

"Daddy, Daddy, Daddy!"

His eyes light up

You can tell she's his world

But he knows if he doesn't change some core habits, he can't guarantee he'll be around for her best years.

The decision is his and his alone.

Will he make the clear and obvious choice?

Fast-forward 20 years...

A girl on her wedding day.

Picture-perfect dress.

The beach in the background.

This should be the happiest day of her life

She has tears in her eyes

But they aren't just tears of joy…

The only man she loves as much as your husband…

…Isn't there to walk her down the aisle

Why?

He couldn't change his habits, had a heart attack and passed away a few years prior.

Open your eyes now ;)

That's what this is about!

Serge is a real person (last name withheld) who inquired with me 5 years ago to the day give or take.

Only to tell me he didn't have the time to commit right now to his health with his work and family commitments.

Unfortunately, I saw a post months later on his Facebook page from his wife, informing everyone Serge died that day at 44 years old, of a heart attack on his bathroom floor.

Leaving behind 3 pre-teen daughters.

Nowadays, they leave a post once a year on his profile, daughters talking to daddy about what they've accomplished that year.

It breaks my heart seeing those, but it reminds me why I do this all the same.

I have two young daughters of my own.

It's not about getting ripped for a magazine cover (though that's a noble goal and I won't judge those who pursue it)

It's about being the best version of you for as many years as you can muster so you're the best parent, provider and human you can be.

It all starts with making a commitment to yourself.

You intuitively know those magic pills, shrink wraps and 30 day challenges aren't sustainable.

Commitment to better habits is the key, not motivation or willpower.

By getting your health handled, you'll...

...Produce more of yourself in work and family

...Amplify resistance to stress and pressure

...Have the energy and vitality to enjoy life at a much higher level.

And yes... of course, look great naked, and feel many years younger than your years.

Life's only one trip around the merry-go-round and you only get one vessel (your body) to ride around in.

Treat it right. Hard decisions now lead to an easy life later. The opposite is true if you cave to immediate gratification right now. So this book aims to help you find your path to the promised land.

THE SCARY STATISTICS

Why are over 30% of Canadians (and 40% of Americans) clinically obese?

We know what to do but have a hard time doing it.

Case in point, we try to take a trip every year to escape winter. One thing I noticed is how out of shape the hotel guests were compared to the locals. It was a stark contrast. And it's always the case.

The protruding turtle-shell belly (in both sexes) I saw everywhere is often a sign of visceral fat accumulation around the organs. This dangerous type of fat has been linked to heart disease, Type 2 diabetes, high cholesterol, certain cancers and stroke.

Mind your own business, Mitch! I know, I know. This is a touchy subject. Let's be clear, I'm speaking in generalities here and not judging anyone individually. But it is my business, because I'm in the fitness business and obesity rates continue to rise despite efforts to reverse this trend.

Why is that? We seemingly know what to do to get into better shape but have a hard time doing it. I'm sure I'll get some hate for this perspective, but I ask you to explore the source within that's causing you to feel offended. If you are 100 percent happy with yourself, this shouldn't create any hate. But, if you're offended, find out why. There might be something there, like there was for me back in 2002.

I'm thankful I got called out by a gym teacher in high school after dry heaving my way through a routine drill. Sometimes we need "tough love" to replace "self love" or change doesn't happen. I don't know if I would've had the motivation to change if I didn't face the reality of my circumstances at 260 pounds that early in life. It took another person to wake me up to the realities of my situation and that was enough spark to start.

This message isn't meant to fill you with guilt, but it is about taking an honest look in the mirror and facing reality. If you're obese like I was, chances are we're shaving years off our lives, and 'life' from our days.

The reality is it's difficult to be healthy and fit at a body mass index (BMI) over 30. The science is clear as the ocean on this one. Literally hundreds of studies have been done on the relationship between BMI and health and they show a reasonably consistent J-shaped relation-ship between BMI and all-cause mortality — the risk of dying from any cause.

People generally have the lowest chance of dying when their BMI is between 20 and 25. There is a progressively higher risk when they're underweight or overweight, and a much higher risk when obese.

BMI is not perfect, but it's what we have that can be easily measured in a doctor's office (and still applies to the majority of people — aside from the one percent of people with high levels of muscle mass rela-tive to body fat).

Yes, I shouldn't judge a book by its cover, and some of those I observed may be mid-journey and taking a well-earned break to enjoy what an all-inclusive resort has to offer, but we know these are the exceptions to the rule.

It's not opinion, it's fact. Worldwide obesity has tripled since 1975 and is one of the leading causes of cancer and cardiovascular disease. Addressing it is not as simple as telling people to eat better and exercise more, I get that. It's a complex disease with multiple layers of challenges.

But, for me, taking some personal responsibility was the first step, and one I'm happy I begrudgingly took back in the day.

At the time, I wasn't a very happy person. In fact, I was miserable. A victim of my circumstances, or so I convinced myself.

But I was convinced that once I got in shape, then it would all fall into place. Of course, that was only one piece of the puzzle. The big wave of happiness I was expecting it to come with wasn't immediate.

And instead of realizing a leaner abdomen was never going to fill that emptiness, I basically doubled down on it.

I thought "well once I have a six pack, it'll all change." This kind of thinking went on for more time than I'd like to admit.

Getting frisked with a chicken breast in my pocket at a sports bar was a low point of my extremism. It was always "once I get to the next level" I'll be happy.

But I started to slowly realize that exterior changes alone were never going to make me happy. They could help me find it, but it still had to come from within.

Because here's the thing: I started to realize the journey was actually going to be the source of happiness — if I let it. By following through on my commitments in the gym, it carried over to other areas of my life.

However, a healthy body led to a healthy mind. I applied the same principles to my career pursuits and more opportunities came my way. Same with relationships. Take care of yourself and put in the time and you attract the outcomes you want. And I held my head up high knowing I was doing the work and that automatically meant people treated me better.

You have to enjoy the journey, because the end result doesn't guarantee more happiness. Don't let the pursuit of your end goal make you overlook all the good that's happening along the way. The residual benefits of a healthier body and mind are the true prizes. Improved health and more energy, patience, confidence and strength are the things that come from doing the work, and they'll happen sooner than you think — once you start. Those go much further than the number on the scale at the end of the day.

SCARY STORY FROM SWIM LESSONS

The other night, amidst the echoes of splashes at our girls' swim lessons, I overheard a conversation I couldn't help but eavesdrop on.

It was about a fellow parent's father, battling for life in the ICU with a cocktail of medications just to keep his heart beating and fluid retention at bay.

It made me pause for a second to reflect. We hustle through our days in an endless pursuit, overlooking the most precious gift we have — our health.

I've been wrestling with sleep issues myself and it's been a journey of ups and downs, as I've shared in this space, with no easy solution. But hearing this story, I realized my problems are small in comparison.

But the reminder I got that night was that health isn't just about looking good or hitting fitness goals. It's about being there for our kids' swim lessons, growing old with our loved ones and living life without the burden of preventable illnesses (not assuming this guy's was, but you get my point!).

Let's not wait for a wake-up call to cherish our health. Let's be grateful for the present, for our body's strength and for every breath we take. Because in the end, what else do we need? It's the foundation of all the memories we cherish and the moments we live for.

IS THAT A CHICKEN
BREAST IN YOUR POCKET?

It was a sunny June afternoon circa 2009 and I was heading to a UFC event with a few buddies. We got there early to take in the festivities, and I figured I would go for at least six hours without a proper meal. So, naturally, I packed a chicken breast smothered with peanut butter in my pocket.

Unfortunately, the bouncer at the door frisked me, found the chicken breast, and inquired, "WTF is that?" I explained my predicament — and the muscle loss that would surely follow — and he said I was mostly at risk for salmonella and suggested I eat it right then and there or he'd toss it out.

Long story short, I had to force down some dry chicken in front of a line-up of UFC fans. Hardcore. So what am I trying to tell you with this trip down memory lane? In the early days of my fitness journey as a young and naive Mitch, I replaced one obsession (junk food and video games) with another (extreme weight lifting and healthy eating) instead of taking a balanced approach.

I withdrew myself further from the world, measuring every morsel of food that went into my mouth, refusing to eat dinner with my family and avoiding social gatherings so I could maximize my deep sleep.

It took a while to come to the realization that I was wasting some of the best years of my life to try to maximize my results in the gym. My approach now focuses on balance and moderation (in fact, I get

better results now that I've loosened the reins a bit) and that's 15 ultimately what my clients want, too.

So I want to let you know that you can reach your fat loss goals while
enjoying barbecues and beers. This book is going to show you how.

THE LAW OF RED VELVET CAKE

My guilty pleasure. Specifically, the one a local iconic restaurant, Salisbury House, makes.

The icing.. to die for.

The melt in your mouth filling... orgasmic.

But The Law of Red Velvet Cake keeps me honest.

It goes like this:

If the cake doesn't get into my car, it doesn't get home.

And if it doesn't get home, it doesn't get in my mouth.

And if it doesn't get in my mouth, it doesn't contribute to belly fat.

You feel me?

If the temptation is in the house, you are going to indulge eventually.

White knuckling it with willpower alone isn't a winning formula.

This rule can be applied to your guilty pleasure.

What is it you can't help yourself around? Let me know in the comments.

(And then make sure it isn't staring at you from the pantry except on special occasions)

WHAT'S TO BLAME FOR WEIGHT GAIN?

Is it carbs? The carb insulin model (CIM) of obesity, originally proposed by Dr. David Ludwig and popularized by the likes of Gary Taubes and Jason Fung, would have you think so.

The CIM basically states that people don't get obese from eating too many calories, they get obese from chronically elevated insulin (from carbohydrate intake) which traps fat in fat cells, making it inaccessible to the rest of the body to be used as energy.

Calories 101

Before we get to the data comparing diets, let's discuss some basics. Calories are a measurement of the amount of energy within a food. The 3,500-calorie rule is generally understood to equal one pound of body weight change.

In layman's terms, if an individual has a goal of losing one pound per week, they will have to reduce calorie intake by 500 calories per day (500 x 7 = 3,500) to achieve one pound of weight loss. But one pound per week can look very different depending on how it's achieved. The individual who strength-trains and eats sufficient protein while reducing calories largely will lose fat while someone cutting calories and nothing else may lose a good percentage of muscle.

What the research shows

How does the CIM stack up against conventional calorie restriction? As with anything, you can generally find something to support your bias and that's no different here.

We have a mountain of research studies that compare low-fat to low-carb strategies, when the two most important variables, calories and protein, are accounted for. In a 2017 meta analysis, researchers found no net benefit to low-carb diets, and perhaps a slight advantage to the opposite, high-carb, low-fat diets.

A 2021 Ludwig study leaned in favour of low-carb diets on the basis of higher daily energy expenditure. Ludwig's lab found more calories burned in low-carb dieters, but it didn't lead to more losses of body fat. In response, other researchers called into question the methods used to measure energy expenditure, as without fat losses to show for it, can we really take much from this finding?

What should you do?

Much is made of the low-carb vs. low-fat debate, but based on the evidence we have today, it does not seem to make a difference.

Both low-fat and low-carb diets (and everything in between) appear to be equally effective for fat loss so long as protein and calories are equated between diets.

Low-fat diets work by reducing fat so you eat fewer calories by default. Low-carb diets work by reducing carbohydrates so you eat fewer calories by default. Intermittent fasting works by restricting your eating to one eight-hour period each day so you eat less calories by default. You get where I'm going with this. It all comes down to energy balance: if you're gaining weight, you're eating more calories than you're expending and vice versa if you're losing.

The best diet is one you can stick to. If you enjoy a ketogenic diet and can sustain it for a long time, go for it. I personally prefer focusing on the fundamentals. Case in point, we just awarded our "Client of the Quarter" vacation giveaway to Sean, who lost 108 pounds in a year.

Last year he noticed he was getting winded going up flights of stairs and didn't have the energy to keep up with his hectic work and travel demands — nor to be at his best for his family!

Sean had read my *Free Press* column and the simple message resonated. Despite a healthy dose of skepticism, he took the leap.

Physical changes aside, his health markers one year on are the most positive developments:

- Body mass index BMI dropped 15 points

- Blood pressure dropped from 160/90 to 120/60

- Resting heart rate fell from 80 beats per minute to 60

- Over 30 inches in circumference off his midsection (not a misprint)

So, how did Sean do it? The process to make this happen is simple on paper.

Start with the big 5 basics this book is based on and we'll get into the nitty gritty for you in the pages ahead:

1. Walk 8,000-10,000 steps daily by tracking your movement with wearable technology (even your smartphone does this by default!).

2. Drink two to four liters of water daily and track your intake with a calibrated jug or water system.

3. Eat mostly whole foods with 80 percent of your meals prepared at home, not purchased at a restaurant or drive-thru. You'll probably need to track your calories and proteins if eating healthy has gotten you nowhere in the past.

4. Strength-train at least three times a week for 30 minutes. The role exercise plays is primarily in maintaining muscle here, so choose wisely. It's not high-intensity interval training (HIIT), boot camps or circuit workouts that serve this role best.

5. Get seven-plus hours of sleep most nights by committing to a set bedtime.

If you were able to implement these five habits at 80 per cent consistency, I'm confident that in three months...

- You could be down 20 pounds — or more — when you step on the scale;

- You could be eating carbs — every single day! — and making your keto friends jealous;

- You could feel like you're not working out that hard and still seeing better results than with those boot camps.

But navigating life's challenges, staying consistent and customizing it to yourself is the tricky part. If you're willing to do the legwork, you'll understand what matters and have all the tools to keep the weight of

FEAR SELLS
(HERE'S HOW TO
TELL FACT FROM FICTION)

Everywhere I look online people say "seed oils" will destroy your health. But what does the research really say?

And how do you know who — and what — to believe when you read an article on the internet?

Fear sells. When you make fear-based comments and claims, people notice. And "seed oils cause obesity, inflammation, cancer and will kill you if you eat them" is that exact kind of nonsense.

It's just the latest in a long line of "nutritional boogeymen" since the obesity epidemic came into full swing in the early 1980s.

At first, the boogeyman was saturated fat and cholesterol.

In 1984, *Time* magazine went with a cover featuring frowny-face sunny-side-up eggs and bacon under the headline *Cholesterol: And Now the Bad News*, and everyone ditched bacon and eggs for a while. Fat was making us fat and clogging our arteries, or so we were told.

But of course, over time we realized it made little impact either way.

The next nutritional boogeyman was sugar, and eventually all carbs. After all, eating less fat didn't work, so the answer must be sugar, right? We're eating too many carbs, which is causing our insulin to spike, and insulin is a "storage hormone." (This theory is called the insulin hypothesis, and it's had plenty of holes poked in it in recent years, by the way.)

So, *Time* magazine went in the other direction, and came out with another cholesterol-related cover in 2014. This time, the headline *Eat Butter: Scientists labeled fat the enemy. Why they were wrong* ran above a photograph of an artistically sculpted curl of butter.

And like clockwork, all the food companies said, "shoot, nobody wants to buy our low-fat products any longer! We need to make low-carb products, because carbs are bad!"

And our grocery store shelves were bombarded with low-carb cookies, gluten-free cakes and Atkins-approved muffins.

And of course... it didn't work (yet again). And since obesity rates are still rising, we need another boogeyman.

Sugar consumption has plummeted in the United States over the last decade but our weight and waistlines have expanded at the same rates as before.

Clearly, we haven't pinpointed the proper boogeyman, right?

Now enter seed oils. Common seed oils include canola oil, sunflower oil and safflower oil.

Sometimes, chemical solvents are used to extract the oils as well. This association with "chemicals" is what makes seed oils a prime target to scare people away. People see the words "chemicals" and "processed" (which seed oils are), and the appeal to logical fallacy is difficult to overcome (just like with "artificial" sweeteners).

Seed oils are also high in Omega-6 fatty acids, which scares people, since the Omega-3 to Omega-6 fatty acid ratio needs to be kept in check.

The biggest reason seed oils have been deemed "bad" is because of their association with processed and fried foods.

Processed foods are created to taste delicious. It's tough to lose weight if you're regularly eating junk food like cakes, candy and potato chips. But you already knew that, right? You were never supposed to eat most of your foods from a bag or a box with a barcode. But unfortunately, our world is set up to do just that.

The question remains, is it about the seed oils themselves, or is it the excess calories that come along with eating processed foods?

Even before I started coaching others, I didn't want to know the nitty-gritty scientific facts behind protocols. I just wanted to know what mattered to the average person so I could make it work in layman's terms. Give me the *Cliff's Notes* — that was my motto — and that's what I do for my clients as well.

Because of this, I need to know who to trust, especially in the world of nutrition, which many people treat like religion.

Back in the early 2000s when I was learning how to get fit myself, I came across some dubious information, and took it as gospel.

I fell hook, line and sinker into the "carbs are bad" rhetoric that was running wild online. I went "keto" before it was even a thing.

Did I lose weight? Yep, I sure did, but I also lost muscle, my libido (not cool for a 20-something guy, lol), and kept getting sick (some of that surely would've happened with a crash diet higher in carbs, as well).

I was obsessive about not eating carbs and I was positive that eating them made you fat. Because that's exactly what "everyone said" online. Sound familiar? This is the exact same thing people are saying about seed oils right now.

It wasn't until I sought out trustworthy sources of information that I started to realize I was falling for the fads.

I spent that next year some 18 years ago taking the PN1 course on nutrition, going back to university for night classes, and I hired a coach of my own. I had to find unbiased practitioners and follow their lead.

What is an "unbiased practitioner?" It's a coach or figure who uses nuance when they speak. They never spout absolutes such as "if you eat this one thing, it will destroy your health."

If you listen to "Carnivore Carl" from Twitter, who sells "Carnivore coaching," of course Carnivore Carl will tell you things that fit his narrative.

Every year, as the temperatures rose, so did the number on the scale. Then one fateful summer in my mid 20s, I decided to break free from this cycle and just commit to the basics. I found if I had these foundational five habits in my arsenal — and I applied them near daily — I could mix in fun and still focus on fitness.

Habit 1: H$_2$O to the rescue

I chugged down not one, not two, but a glorious three liters of water every day. It helped wash away the cravings and kept me energized all summer long.

Habit 2: Walking Wonderland

Ah, the joy of walking! I made it my mission to clock in those magical 8,000-10,000 steps every day. Walking became my escape, my time to recharge, and an opportunity to get out while the weather was good.

Habit 3: Get Your Sleep

Sleep is the foundation of your entire fitness plan. Without it, it's hard to adhere to other fundamentals.

Habit 4: Pumping iron

Speaking of muscles, that fateful summer had a new attraction: strength training! I waved goodbye to hours on the treadmill and hit the weights with gusto.

Habit 5: Calorie control caper

I must admit, I had some "triggers" that led to ice cream, barbecues — you name it! But I embraced the awareness that tracking my portions provided me. I enjoyed those indulgences mindfully, while making sure my overall intake played nice with my goals.

My approach has evolved over the years, but these foundational five habits are the framework. I promise you it makes things a whole lot more enjoyable and sustainable if you choose to do the same.

Let's break these down a little further...

BIG 5 FRAMEWORK

1) H_2O to the rescue

I chugged down not one, not two, but a glorious three liters of water every day. It helped wash away the cravings and kept me energized.

Hydration is another critical component of weight loss and overall health. Drinking adequate water can aid in weight loss by increasing satiety and enhancing metabolic rate. Plus, staying hydrated is essential for proper bodily functions, including digestion and muscle function.

2) Walk This Way

You might be surprised with the impact of walking on your fat-loss journey. Incorporating 8,000-10,000 (don't fixate too much on the number) steps into your daily routine can make a significant difference. Whether you choose to do it all at once or weave those steps in throughout the day, it amounts to approximately 45-60 minutes daily. No small feat. But mini 10-minute walks add up. You can even turn those Zoom meetings or calls into productive walking sessions!

Walking, especially when done regularly, has been shown to contribute significantly to weight loss and overall health. According to Harvard T.H. Chan School of Public Health, walking is not only beneficial for physical health but also for mental well-being. It can lower the risk of chronic diseases and even reduce mortality. Even moderate amounts of walking, like 150 minutes per week, have been associated with a lower risk of early death, which is substantial considering the average American walks about 4,800 steps a day. The benefits increase with more steps but plateau around 7,500 steps per day.

From Mayo Clinic, we learn that incorporating walking into your daily routine can help burn additional calories. A combination of physical activity and dietary changes seems more effective for weight loss than exercise alone. While it's important to balance and avoid overdoing it, walking can be a key component in maintaining weight loss over the long term.

3) Sleep Off The Fat?

It's well-documented that adequate sleep plays a critical role in weight management and overall health. Poor sleep has been linked to weight gain and can affect the hormones that regulate hunger and appetite. Aim for 7-8 hours of quality sleep per night to support your weight loss and health goals.

Several cross-sectional studies have indicated that short sleep duration is associated with obesity and the risk of future weight gain in both adults and children.

One common hypothesis about the connection between weight and sleep involves how sleep affects appetite. While we often think of appetite as simply a matter of stomach grumbling, it's actually controlled by neurotransmitters, which are chemical messengers that allow neurons (nerve cells) to communicate with one another.

The neurotransmitters ghrelin and leptin are thought to be central to appetite. Ghrelin promotes hunger, and leptin contributes to feeling full. The body naturally increases and decreases the levels of these neurotransmitters.

A lack of sleep may affect the body's regulation of these neurotransmitters. In one study, men who got 4 hours of sleep had increased ghrelin and decreased leptin compared to those who got 10 hours of sleep. This dysregulation of ghrelin and leptin may lead to increased appetite and diminished feelings of fullness in people who are sleep deprived.

In addition, several studies have also indicated that sleep deprivation affects food preferences. Sleep-deprived individuals tend to choose foods that are high in calories and carbohydrates.

And how do we lose fat? It's converted to carbon dioxide and water.

If you lose 10 pounds of fat, precisely 8.4 pounds comes out through your lungs and the remaining 1.6 pounds turns into water. In other words, nearly all the weight we lose is exhaled, much of that happens while you're in recovery mode breathing regularly while you sleep!

This surprises just about everyone, but actually, almost everything we eat comes back out via the lungs. Every carbohydrate you digest and nearly all the fats are converted to carbon dioxide and water. The same goes for alcohol.

We all know that getting enough sleep is essential for our health and well-being, but a new study suggests that it's not just about the number of hours we spend in slumber—it's also about the regularity of our sleep patterns.

According to researchers, maintaining an irregular sleep schedule can lead to a shorter life. In particular, better sleep regularity is associated with up to a 48 percent lower risk of all-cause mortality, as high as 39 percent lower risk of cancer mortality, and more than 50 percent lower risk of cardiometabolic mortality.

Irregular sleepers refer to people who go to sleep at different times or consistently shift between different sleep durations. So, if you wildly vary when you sleep and wake or dramatically shift how much you sleep each night, either can potentially cause health issues.

Instead, having a consistent sleep schedule — trying to sleep a similar number of hours, as well as going to bed and waking at a similar time — can have a significant impact on your overall health and longevity.

You can help regulate your sleep by getting sunlight early in the day (this can help reset your internal clock and help you fall asleep earlier), limiting food about 2 to 3 hours before you sleep, and reducing stimulating activities before bedtime, such as using electronic devices or consuming caffeinated beverages. All of these can harm your sleep cycle and make it harder to fall asleep.

In summary, here are some general tips to optimize your sleep hygiene:

- Keep a regular sleep schedule: Big swings in your sleep schedule or trying to catch up on sleep after a week of late nights can cause changes in metabolism and reduce insulin sensitivity

- Sleep in a dark room: Exposure to artificial light while sleeping, such as a TV or bedside lamp, is associated with an increased risk of weight gain and obesity.

- Don't eat right before bed: Eating late may reduce the success of weight loss attempts. But don't go to bed starving, either.

- National Library of Medicine, Biotech Information

- The National Center for Biotechnology Information advances science and health by providing access to biomedical and genomic information.

- Reduce Stress: Chronic stress may lead to poor sleep and weight gain in several ways, including eating to cope with negative emotions

- Be an Early Bird: People with late bedtimes may consume more calories and be at a higher risk for weight gain

4) The Power of the Pump

When it comes to losing weight, it's not just about lowering the number on the scale. We want to lose body fat while maintaining muscle mass. This is where weightlifting comes in. Engaging in weightlifting sessions three to four times a week can work wonders for your transformation. In fact, research has shown weightlifting helps preserve muscle while shedding fat. It's about quality, not just quantity.

Strength Training for Weight Loss: A study highlighted in ScienceDaily reveals that strength training can effectively reduce body fat. The research underscores the importance of considering overall body composition rather than just focusing on weight. Strength training offers numerous benefits, including the improvement of lean mass and muscle quality, and it can also contribute to fat loss, a benefit traditionally associated with aerobic exercises.

Muscle Mass and Metabolic Rate: Another study from the Current Sports Medicine Reports indicates that resistance training can lead to an increase in lean weight and resting metabolic rate while reducing fat weight. This supports the idea that strength training is not just about building muscle, but it also plays a crucial role in improving metabolic health and aiding in fat loss.

Weight-training strategy: I'm often asked about the "best" training programs. Instead of focusing solely on one-size-fits-all, let's delve deeper into strategy. The "just-one-more" mindset is a game-changer.

In each workout, strive for just one more rep, set or small increase in weight. It might seem like a minor step, but across multiple workouts, it adds up to substantial progress. This approach helps you maintain consistent growth and improvement over time.

Progressive overload and structured workouts: Building a lean and strong body isn't about random workouts thrown together haphazardly. It's about a strategic approach that involves progressive overload — increasing your strength and reps over time. Muscle preservation and growth thrive on structured routines. Instead of chasing the latest fitness trends, focus on the basics that have stood the test of time. Those exercises are the ones that fit nicely into movement patterns you'll need in your everyday life, which include:

- Upper-body push: bench press and push ups

- Upper-body pull: rows and pull-ups

- Hip hinge: deadlifts, good mornings or kettlebell swings

- Squats: front squats, back squats or goblet squats

- Loaded carry: farmer's walk

- Everything else: single-leg exercises and core exercises

The journey to success: The path to effective fat loss isn't paved with shortcuts or quick fixes. It's about making conscious, sustainable choices that align with your goals. Small steps lead to significant changes, and progress is your constant companion. Visualize the progress you'll make a year from now — lifting more weight, performing more reps — and envision the transformation it'll bring to your body and mindset.

Remember, it's not about dramatic shifts or drastic sacrifices. It's about consistency, balance and embracing the journey with open arms. If you're prepared to dedicate yourself to these steps, you're well on your way to a healthier, leaner you.

Almost everything you need to know about strength training is included in this chapter.

That's probably the exact opposite info you've been fed by mainstream fitness over the years. The problem with most "mainstream" fitness is the randomness of it.

Pop into your local boot camp gym, turn on your Tonal app or fire up your Peloton and do whatever suits your fancy that day. You leave exhausted and accomplished. Done.

One problem: sweating doesn't equal success. Changing your body doesn't happen by accident. Exercise in all forms is great, and you should do any type of exercise you enjoy. But if you want to lose fat, tone up, boost metabolism and improve bone density, the secret to success is structured strength training.

It's the type of training that may look a bit repetitive, but builds upon itself over time. Heck, even the Peloton instructors didn't build their bodies with Peloton workouts alone. (I love my Peloton for mixing in some movement, so I feel like a cheating spouse here, but it's the truth.)

So, what's the solution? Make sure your plan adheres to these main tenets:

— Train three to five days per week with weights as your foundation and mix in movement however you want

— Use a program that gives you enough volume per muscle group, per week (10-20 sets per muscle group, per week, depending on goals and stage of development)

— Track your performance improvements (more reps, or a bit more weight)

— Stick to one program for at least eight to 12 weeks

Problem: Where do you start? Well, that's what we're discussing today — so strap in!

The seven steps to building the perfect workout program

1) Training intensity: If you aren't training hard enough, nothing else matters. This doesn't mean lifting the heaviest weight possible until you can't do another rep and injure yourself. A good rule of thumb is to challenge yourself with a weight that gets you anywhere between one to three reps shy of failing — the point where you can't complete another rep with good form.

So, if you can lift a weight for a maximum of 10 reps with a given weight, anywhere between seven and nine reps will be stimulating enough for muscle growth to occur.

2) Progressive overload: To grow and get stronger, you need to increase the demands placed on your body during successive work-outs.

While there are a number of ways you can implement progressive overload, the simplest is to focus on lifting more weight or completing more reps than you did in the previous session.

Finally, just remember you won't always be able to make progress every time you train, especially once you're past the beginner stage. Every small improvement makes a difference at that point. Some weeks you'll make progress, other weeks you might not. That's fine as long as progress is happening over time.

3) Training volume: Volume is the number of working sets per muscle group, per week. The latest research on the topic suggests anywhere between 12 and 20 sets per muscle group, per week, is likely optimal for muscle growth.

That said, studies only tell us about group averages and you, as an individual, might need more or less volume than what's stated above.

For example, a beginner might start with 10 sets per muscle group, per week, and work their way up to 12 sets over time.

Finally, what matters most is the effort you put forth. Doing a bunch of extra sets with poor form is counterproductive here. Get in, work hard and get out.

4) Reps: All rep ranges can build muscle and tone as long as you're getting close to failure, so you can use a wide range of reps in your training.

However, if the goal is muscle growth, most of your training should occur in the six- to 12-rep range. It's not because there's anything inherently special about this rep range, but constantly training with lower reps (one to five) means lifting heavy weights really close to your maximum that can increase the risk of injury and generally leave you feeling more beat up.

Doing too much high-rep training can increase fatigue and recovery time, and form can start to break down the longer a set goes.

The six- to 12-rep range is a nice rule of thumb for most exercises, but there's a time and place for going lower or higher.

5) Rest times: The research as a whole tends to favour longer rest periods for muscle and strength gains. Wow, I know — you're pressed for time already! This is where boot camps that have you going non-stop fall short. Longer rest times give your body a chance to clear out

waste, replenish ATP (Adenosine triphosphate, which is needed for strength and muscular contractions), and allow you to give it your all at the next step.

That said, longer rest periods seem more important for multi-joint "compound" movements, while you could probably get away with shorter rest periods for single-joint "isolation" movements. For compound exercises, think barbell squats and presses, while isolation movements would be cable and dumbbell exercises targeting a single muscle group (for instance, dumbbell curls).

I personally like strategic supersets that act as active rest and minimize the "need" to sit around waiting between sets. This is where you're pairing exercises with opposite movement patterns. Think of a classic push-pull or "front and back" superset. For example, pair biceps curls and triceps extensions, so you don't waste time in the gym, but you do get enough recovery in the non-working muscle to give it your all the next time. The best of both worlds.

The science: Rest intervals of two minutes between sets are sufficient for the machine chest fly (isolation exercise) and three to five minutes for the bench press (compound).

6) Training frequency: How often you train per week seems to matter far less once weekly volume is in the 12-20 sets per muscle range. However, the best way to do this is to split those sets over two workouts, which in turn means better performance at each session.

For instance, if you're aiming for 12 sets per muscle group, per week, I don't like the conventional bodybuilder approach of a "chest day" followed by an "arm day," for instance.

You'll find you're better able to maintain training intensity and performance when spreading volume across the week, such as six sets on Monday and six more on Thursday, versus trying to cram all your volume into one session.

You can then set this up based on the number of days you can work out:

— Three days per week: three full-body workouts, lower/upper/full-body

— Four days per week: lower/upper/lower/upper

— Five days per week: upper/lower/upper/lower/upper "pump" (a more joint-friendly workout of lower weights and more reps)

7) Exercise selection: Don't listen to the free-weight purists who say you're not serious about training if you default to machines. Both free weights (dumbbells and barbells) and machines can build muscle. Furthermore, your body doesn't "see" equipment, it only recognizes intensity and effort. And you can apply intensity with all types of equipment. It's all in how you use it.

Choose exercises you feel confident performing, that you connect with and that allow you to safely progress over time.

If you don't want to barbell squat or can't feel it where you should, use the leg press or dumbbell goblet squat. If you don't want to bench press, do a dumbbell or machine variation.

And if you don't want to do burpees? Good, because they are dumb.

5) The CAP Flexibility Framework

Ever heard the saying, "You are what you eat?" Well, it holds some truth. To effectively manage your weight, it's essential to keep track of what you're consuming. This doesn't mean you have to be obsessive about it — thanks to modern technology, it's easier than ever.

I swear by a simple one-two punch to guarantee fat loss - the CAP Flexibility Framework. **The perfect combination of Calories & Protein unique to you so the fat melts off (yes, even if you have some pizza fit in)**

No more guesswork or wondering why you're not progressing.

So how do you figure out your numbers? When it comes to calories, understanding the basics can be a game-changer. A simple calculation involves multiplying your body weight by a factor of 10-12. This provides you with a calorie "range" to aim for, ensuring consistent fat loss. Additionally, if you're looking not just to lose weight, but to specifically target fat loss, multiply your body weight by a factor of 0.8-1. This will give you a protein goal in grams to strive for each day. This balance ensures you're fuelling your body right and losing sustainably.

(Note: If you want to get more scientific with your numbers based on age, activity levels and goal, grab a free report at www.mitchcalvert. com/calculator)

Based on the research, a focus on calorie control seems to be more effective for weight loss than strategies like intermittent fasting. A study in the Journal of the American Heart Association found that the frequency and size of meals had a stronger impact on weight loss or gain than the timing of meals. Specifically, consuming fewer large and medium-sized meals, and opting for smaller meals, was associated with weight reduction over a six-year period. This finding underscores the importance of total calorie intake as a critical factor in weight management, which aligns with the principle of our Big 5 Framework, "CAP Control"

The Heisenberg Hack?

So, maybe I've sorta convinced you that knowing how much you're eating is more important than what you eat when it comes to weight loss.

And the only way to do that successfully in a world setup to easily over-consume is to track your intake initially.

Tracking is the silver bullet most need, but overlook. This doesn't mean you have to be obsessive about it or do it forever. But thanks to modern technology, it's easier than ever.

Why is this important? Because of the Heisenberg Principle! No, not the infamous character from *Breaking Bad* played by Bryan Cranston. A now deceased German physicist who wisely identified that what gets measured, gets managed.

Here's how it works. Picture this: You've been a cookie fiend for 20 years, inhaling them like there's no tomorrow. Now, you decide it's time for a change. But here's the twist — instead of going cold turkey and battling the guilt and frustration that follows, you just start tracking your cookie intake.

That's it. Count those cookies. Without judgment, track them in an app or by jotting intake down on paper.

Monday: 10 cookies. Tuesday: eight. Wednesday: Oops, 12. Don't beat yourself up — just observe and jot it down.

And here's where our friend Heisenberg comes in with his principle: the act of observing something changes it. By simply being aware of your cookie consumption, you're already on the path to improvement, without sweeping changes, fads or extreme measures.

Guess what happens next? Slowly but surely, those cookie numbers start to drop. Not because you're forcing it, but because awareness is a powerful thing.

"Hmm, I'm eating 1,000 calories worth of cookies, maybe that's excessive and I should cut back a bit?"

A month later: Down to five per day. Another month: Just one or two a day. Before you know it, you're shrugging at the cookie jar, thinking, "Meh, I'm good." And the best part? It was all effortless.

So, give the Heisenberg hack a try. Track it, don't attack it.

THE SECRETS SECTION

I hope you've realized the basics make the biggest difference. That's what the first half of this book was all about. But there's a time and place for secrets, so that's what we're going to give you over the next few chapters. Let's dive in.

FAT LOSS DRUGS

Drugs such as Ozempic and Zepbound have revolutionized the treatment of obesity, helping people lose significant amounts of weight without surgery.

Zepbound, containing the active compound tirzepatide, recently entered the United States market. It appears to be a step above its predecessors such as Ozempic, so it's creating some buzz.

The drugs' primary role is to reduce food cravings and appetite. They can also delay gastric emptying, which is the time it takes for food to move through the stomach, so you hit and sustain that full feeling longer than normal.

Appetite can be a major deterrent for many dieters looking to shed pounds. For some, their appetite is ravenous with the slightest calorie drop and no amount of willpower helps. No doubt there's a genetic component at play here. Plus, being overweight and overfed for a long time can break some of the internal hardwiring that regulates how much we eat.

As effective as these medications are, they have their drawbacks. They are pricey, aren't covered by insurance for weight-loss purposes in Canada (just Ozempic is approved for Type 2 diabetes) and they can also have side effects, like nausea and vomiting, stomach pain, and, more rarely, stomach paralysis, pancreatitis and bowel obstructions.

The side effects can be taxing, especially as people first begin the medications. Feeling like you have the flu, even for a short time, was enough to lead to modest dropout rates in studies. Some patients just don't want to deal with injecting themselves indefinitely, either, even if it's just once per week.

Plus, there is not yet robust data on what happens when people take the drugs for decades. Ozempic and Zepbound all belong to a single class of drugs that have been on the market for less than 20 years, so the long-term effects of staying on them for life isn't exactly known.

Buzz around Zepbound

Developed by Eli Lilly, this drug has shown promising results in clinical trials, significantly impacting weight management. A study tracking 670 individuals over 36 weeks showed, on average, they shed 20 per-cent of their body weight during that period.

But it wasn't all good news. The study divided participants after the initial 36-week period. Half continued with Zepbound for another year, while the rest were given a placebo. Those who continued with the medication saw an additional weight loss of 5.5 per cent. Those who were switched to the placebo, however, gained back 14 percent of their body weight on average (of the 20 per cent originally lost). Those on the placebo also tended to have higher cholesterol, blood sugar and blood pressure than they did while taking the medication, which was probably due to a reversal in weight gain and eating habits.

This confirms other research that suggests people seeking weight-loss medication may have to stay on it for the foreseeable future — potentially, for the rest of their lives — if they want to keep the weight off. One study published last April in the journal *Diabetes, Obesity and Metabolism* showed one year after discontinuing use of semaglutide (the active ingredient in Ozempic), participants regained two-thirds of the weight they lost while on the drug.

Quality over quantity

Another downside is the "quality" of the weight lost. Two separate clinical trials for semaglutide showed roughly 40 per cent of the total weight loss experienced by patients was lean body mass (muscle), not just fat.

Though there's limited research so far, I'd suggest you could reverse these negative outcomes (muscle loss and weight regain after ceasing use) by developing the proven strategies that support weight-loss maintenance. Such as strength training, cardio, eating whole foods and taking in a sufficient amount of protein. The same losses of lean muscle are common in dieters who lose weight quickly through unsustainable fads. Your body will "eat up" muscle along with fat if you don't give your muscles a reason to stick around.

And we know not all weight loss is healthy. While shedding excess fat — and in particular, visceral fat — has a multitude of beneficial effects on health, shedding lean mass, which includes muscle and bone, is associated with poorer health and reduced lifespan.

The goal of any program should be to increase the body's overall proportion of muscle — while dropping fat to healthy ranges. As we've discussed, muscle mass is critical to living a long, healthy life. It's not just about keeping our body fat in healthy ranges. Research suggests weight training just once or twice per week reduces mortality risk by 40 per cent compared to people who don't strength-train.

So you cannot rely solely on Zepbound or any weight-loss drug — they can't do the work for you, they just put you in a position to do the work with less self-sabotage.

In a perfect world, should you explore the use of one of these drugs, you would focus on instilling the aforementioned habits built to last while using the medication to support adherence.

Ultimately, you can't get and stay fit without building and maintaining the habits of a fit person. Nothing works until you embrace that reality. But drugs like Ozempic and Zepbound — assuming you can tolerate the side effects and cost — may help you get started and keep going once you do.

I must stress that the medical information in this chapter is provided as an informational resource only, and is not to be used or relied upon for any diagnostic or treatment purpose. This information should not be used as a substitute for professional diagnosis and treatment.

Please consult your health-care provider before making any health-related decisions and for guidance regarding any specific medical condition. Physicians are tasked with balancing the side effects and potential risks against the severe health issues accompanying untreated obesity.

HOT & COLD THERAPY -
ALL SIZZLE NO STEAK?

You see it everywhere on social media. Fitfluencers, bodybuilders, MMA athletes, and maybe even your neighbour — everyone is immersing themselves in tubs filled with ice or cold water, or hopping into home saunas. You can't scroll very far without seeing a post. But is the hype real?

Chilling facts

Ice baths involve submerging oneself in uncomfortably cold water and posting about it on Instagram. Because the cold plunge doesn't count if it isn't documented on social media. I kid. Sorta. The proposed benefits include easing muscle soreness and speeding up muscle recovery, while providing a mood boost. However, the science behind these claims is mixed.

Pros:

Reduced muscle soreness: Studies have found modest positive effects on perceived muscle soreness, especially in athletes like rugby players and MMA fighters.

Improved recovery: Some athletes report quicker recovery post-exercise, potentially aiding in performance. But the science is mixed here as well.

Improved mental boost: Deliberate cold exposure is known to cause an increased flow of epinephrine (a.k.a. adrenaline) and norepinephrine (a.k.a. noradrenaline), making us feel more alert. This may have the most measurable benefit.

Building resilience and grit: This is a hard one to measure, but by facing small uncomfortable tasks, such as an ice-cold shower every morning, Dr. Andrew Huberman suggests you exert what is known as "top-down control" over deeper brain centres that build what we know as resilience and grit.

In other words, deliberate cold exposure is great training for the mind to do hard things.

Metabolism: This one is overblown. It has been shown to convert "white" fat to brown or beige, which is more metabolically active (to prevent you from freezing!) but a salad goes much further than whatever your shower head can do. You burn some marginal calories to increase core body temperature, but it won't help you lose fat if the rest of your plan falls flat.

Cons:

Questionable muscle repair, growth: A study led by Maastricht University researchers revealed cold-water immersion might decrease protein generation in muscles, which is crucial for muscle growth and repair.

While it can potentially help with the recovery and make you feel better, the question is whether the trade-off is worth it. If your goal is to maximize muscle growth, you might want to avoid cold exposure, post workout.

If muscle growth isn't your primary goal, research suggests cold water immersion seems to be fine and may somewhat help boost recovery and performance. Keep in mind cold-water immersion cannot replace the fundamentals — sleep, training, stress management and nutrition — and should only be viewed as a minor tool in your toolbox.

Limited long-term benefits: There's no substantial evidence ice baths improve long-term athletic performance.

Time and comfort: Preparing and taking an ice bath is not only time-consuming but also uncomfortable. Start with a daily cold shower and see if it gives you a boost before investing in a permanent fixture in your backyard.

A quick summary:

Muscle recovery? Science says the benefits might be more of a drip than a splash.

Weight-loss wizardry? Not so fast! Your salad works harder than your shower head.

Inflammation gone? Well, it's more of a maybe than a definitely.

But here's the kicker — I dig them. Why? One word: energy. There's nothing like an icy plunge or a chilly shower to kick-start your day. It's like a caffeine boost without the coffee.

Steaming with speculation

Saunas involve short exposures to high temperatures and are often touted for their relaxing effects and potential health benefits. Despite their popularity, the benefits need more scientific backing.

Cardiovascular function: Regular sauna use may improve cardiovascular function, including endothelium-dependent dilation and lowering blood pressure.

Research shows sauna-bathing may help lower your risk of heart disease. One study followed 2,300 sauna-bathers for 20 years and found the participants who visited the sauna more frequently (four to seven times a week) had lower death rates from heart disease and stroke.

Reduced morbidity and mortality: Frequent sauna use might protect against cardiovascular and neurodegenerative diseases and reduce overall morbidity and mortality.

In addition to lowering cardiovascular-related mortality, sauna use may have benefits for overall longevity. For example, using the sauna two to three times per week is associated with 24 percent lower all-cause mortality and using the sauna four to seven times per week is associated with 40 per cent lower all-cause mortality.

Sauna use is also associated with a lower risk of age-related conditions like Alzheimer's disease.

People who used the sauna two to three times per week had a 20 per cent lower risk of Alzheimer's, and those who used the sauna four to seven times per week had a 60 per cent lower risk of Alzheimer's, compared to men that used the sauna once a week.

Some of the longevity benefits of sauna use may have to do with an increase in heat-shock proteins, which is one of the protective adaptive responses to heat stress. Heat-shock proteins have been shown to prevent and slow the progression of neurodegenerative diseases like Alzheimer's and Parkinson's, slow human muscle atrophy, and are associated with human longevity.

Some of the positive benefits of the sauna on heart health may have to do with similar physiological changes that also occur during physical exercise. However, they shouldn't be considered a worthy replacement for regular exercise.

A quick summary:

Heart health hero: Regular sauna sessions may improve cardiovascular function. Think better blood flow and possibly lower blood pressure — it's like a workout for your heart, without the sweat! (Well, a different kind of sweat.)

Stress buster: Relaxing in a sauna can be a fantastic way to unwind and relieve stress. It's your personal zen zone!

Longevity lifeline? Some studies suggest frequent sauna use might help reduce the risk of cardiovascular and neurodegenerative diseases. Talk about heating up your health.

Hydration hazard: Watch out for dehydration! Saunas can get extremely hot, so staying hydrated is key.

Heat overload: Sauna use isn't for everyone. If you have certain health conditions, it's best to consult with your doctor beforehand. Safety first, sauna second.

Science still simmering: While there are promising studies, the sauna isn't a cure-all. The long-term impact on health, especially for athletic performance, is still under investigation.

* * *

While ice baths and saunas may offer some benefits, their impact pales in comparison to more established health practices.

STAYING CONSISTENT?

So, there you have it, there's no getting around the requirement to eat right, exercise and prioritize your sleep and recovery.

I think almost everyone can relate to the difficulty of doing that consistently. For two weeks, you're dialed in. You're eating better and following a workout program and it goes great... for two weeks. You avoid the crap food and indulgences... for two weeks. You don't miss any workouts... for two weeks. All goes well... for two weeks.

Then the novelty wears off and old habits return. No one's checking on you so you hit snooze and skip a workout or two. Then you stop planning ahead and end up defaulting to drive-thrus and delivery apps again. Only to end up back in that vicious cycle to nowhere. On and off the wagon, rinse and repeat.

Then you say it again... "Nothing works for me." Your self-confidence erodes and you search for some new solution that'll serve you better next time. But the truth is nothing works for you until you work at it. So how do you go from stuck to sustaining next time? There are two things you're missing:

1. 'Be it before you are it'

Better than "Fake it till you make it" (which is based on a façade you can't sustain), you need to fundamentally become the new version of yourself in mindset, habits and belief before the outcome you seek will become reality.

You can't be fit with crappy habits, meaning there's no way you get the desired outcome without ditching some of the habits that lead in the opposite direction — alcohol after dinner every night, skipping the gym, chips and Netflix, and so on.

2. Power of the hive

Look around and ask yourself if there are people in your corner supporting or calling you out when you need it.

By paying for mentoring and coaching you can "borrow" education, experience and even belief from those around you. It's a way to break through your own perceived limits and sustain through the lows.

Of course, the wrinkle is you still have to implement the plan and stick it out. Most people have unrealistic expectations of how fast things should happen for them. That sets them up to fail. Heck, I've been there. After I had my big "weight" wake-up call in my early 20s, tipping the scales at 260 pounds, I wanted to lose every pound as fast as possible.

That didn't happen. That first year ended up being a rude awakening. Why? Because things didn't happen as fast as I thought they would. I had expectations of being down 60 pounds in six months or less.

Instead, I lost 10 only to gain back 10, rinse and repeat, jumping from one quick fix to the next. So when I only lost 10 or so pounds in that first year, give or take, I considered that a failure. But I was 10 pounds further along than I would've been if I did nothing.

In fact, I was adding at least five to 10 pounds per year prior, so it was a 20-pound swing. But I didn't see it that way.

I remember talking with my first fat-loss coach about it the next year. One of the things he helped me see was that I had unrealistic expectations about how fast I was going to build my body.

"Dude, you've been living on chicken fingers and fries, playing video games for six years, it's not going to take six weeks or even six months to undo that."

He wasn't wrong. With his help, I committed a lot better that next year and lost most of the weight over the next 12 months.

I eventually realized the true prize was all the residual benefits that came along with a commitment to fitness.

By committing to the process of getting healthier, I found it changed my work ethic for the better. I was more productive each day. It gave me a better outlook and my mood and mental health made a complete 180.

Frankly, before embracing fitness, my weight was holding me back. I remember eating my lunch in the bathroom in high school if I didn't see the one familiar face I considered a "friend" because I was so lacking in confidence.

Changing the way I saw the world — from a more positive place, not so much a victim — ended up being more valuable than the changes I saw in the mirror. Losing weight and feeling great was the launch pad for the life I live today.

Did getting in shape make me happy? Not by itself. It provided the spark for more contentment and internal satisfaction.

But gradually I've realized happiness is there when you remove the sense of something missing in your life. We constantly walk around thinking, "I need this," or "I need that," trapped in this pursuit that has no end.

And once we get "that" we fill the void in pursuit of another "that" without celebrating the previous "that" we accomplished.

Happiness is the state when nothing is missing. When nothing is missing, your mind shuts down and stops running into the past or future to regret something or to plan something. Feel free to disagree and email me a counterpoint (like you all do when I celebrate carbohydrates in this chapter!).

I rarely achieve this state as I find myself wanting the next thing, too, and the next thing gives me a sense of purpose.

I hate getting complacent, so it's not for me to be in this mindset all the time. But there's probably a middle ground where you can be perfectly content with where you're at while striving for more to fully reach your potential.

Again, it's different for everybody. To me, happiness is not about positive thoughts. It's about the absence of desire, especially the absence of desire for external things.

The fewer desires I can have, the more I can accept the current state of things, the less the voice in my head is fearing the future or stewing in the past. The more present I am, the happier and more content I will be.

Happiness to me is not suffering, not desiring, not thinking too much about the future or the past, and really embracing the present moment and the reality of what is, and the way it is.

When you think of it, this is how toddlers operate.

They're generally pretty happy (meltdowns aside) because they are immersed in the environment and the moment, not stuck in their head, staring at a phone or regretting the past or desiring a different future. Try to model them and see what happens.

MOMENTUM OVER MOTIVATION

I get asked all the time: "How do you stay motivated?"

Fact: I don't. But I work at it.

Motivation is like a muscle — the more you flex it, the stronger it becomes.

But it doesn't stick around forever, and this chapter aims to help you do the work, whether you feel like it all the time or not.

Anytime I'm feeling "in a rut" with my diet and training, this is what I do.

First, I check myself and realize I'm letting the inner voice in my head win.

Second, feelings aren't facts. You feel unmotivated or tired, but that doesn't mean you can't do the work. You must operate on autopilot here to stay consistent.

Feelings come and go. It's OK to feel. But your feelings don't dictate whether the work gets done or not.

If I only trained or stuck to my meals on days I felt like doing it — I'd be back at 250-plus pounds where I spent the better part of my 20s.

Stay in control by having systems: a structured way of eating with room for some fun; the 10-minute rule to get workouts started; sleep and movement routines.

But what do you do if you're just trying to start?

Every time we make a choice outside our default programming, our subconscious mind will attempt to pull us back to the familiar by creating mental resistance. Old habits die hard!

That "resistance" you'll face can take the form of cyclical (and cynical) thoughts, such as "I screwed up, let's quit," or physical symptoms, such as anxiety or frustration.

This is your subconscious communicating to you that it's uncomfortable with these proposed changes. You want to embrace that as a necessary part of change. Everyone feels, but those who succeed push through anyway.

I've put together a list of proven ways to build motivation into your healthy habits backed by science.

1. Make it fun! Try a new recipe. Do a new workout. Listen to your favourite music. Pair your new habit with something you already enjoy doing (walking on the treadmill while watching Netflix, for example).

2. Set a goal that gets you psyched. Sign up for a challenge. Go for a weekend hike. Put some skin in the game, because without a time and financial commitment there is no commitment.

3. Make it part of your routine. Park farther away from your destination. Take the stairs. Go for a lunchtime walk outside. Work out as soon as you wake up in the morning. Hit the grocery store first thing on a weekend morning.

4. Create a journal. Document your progress: What did you do today that was great? What are you planning to do tomorrow? Write it down — and also note how you feel about it.

5. Set up a reward system! Internal rewards: Be sure to tell yourself "good job" every time you follow through on your commitments to yourself. (It really does matter.) External rewards: Set milestones and then reward yourself (new shoes, upgraded gear, book a massage) for reaching them.

6. Build a solid support and accountability circle. Find a supportive friend or group that will keep you moving forward. Working with a coach is invaluable here!

7. Motivate somebody else. Motivating others is incredibly motivating for you. How do I know? Well, let's just say I'm writing this chapter and it's getting me psyched about my own workout and meal-prep plan, for example.

8. Start the day off right. When you start your morning with a healthy meal or workout, it can set the tone for the entire day.

I have been asked to share some motivational tactics you can use to stay consistent. How can you address the mental part of pursuing fitness?

Well, for one thing, I don't "motivate" my clients. That word is overused. As I said off the top, motivation comes and goes and isn't something you want to rely on.

Momentum is the word to embrace here. If a client is struggling with consistency, it's almost never because of a lack of motivation. The lack of motivation is just the surface-level stuff, but there's usually something else going on.

Typically, it's one of two things (or both):

1. They think they're not making progress, even when they are, which results in a lack of motivation to continue.

2. They think they need to be perfect and if they're not, the "screw it" attitude rears its head and they self-sabotage, making it worse.

The most common example of this is if a client is only focusing on their scale weight. This is where I come in and help by providing objective feedback and reminding them of the bigger picture.

I'll explain why scale fluctuations happen and why the scale isn't always a good indicator of progress. I'll show them their progress photos or point out the changes in their body measurements.

Or, potentially, we'll give them constructive criticism on what's likely causing a slowdown in their results. This helps them see they're still getting stronger and feeling better, and this can help them get out of their head and see the bigger picture, which increases motivation.

Perfection isn't the goal — consistency is. Often a client will have one bad day of eating and feel they've ruined all their progress. I'll explain that unless they consumed tens of thousands of calories, it's impossible to "ruin all their progress," and assure them that as long as they get back on track the following day, their daily average intake will balance out.

You should know that coaching is a collaboration, not a dictatorship. It's designed to help you save yourself by giving you the system and support. I don't expect perfection from my clients, I just expect them to do the best they can.

BEYOND THE MEAL PLANS AND MOVEMENTS

Fat loss is about so much more than counting calories and lifting weights (thankfully, or I'd be pretty bored by now having talked about this stuff for more than a decade).

The work between the ears matters most. When you marry belief in yourself with a clear vision of where you want to go, all you need to do is action a plan long enough to get you there. You can, quite literally, paint the picture and be Bob Ross, bringing your dream body to life (perm optional).

So take the time to imagine who you can become, what you've done and how you'll look and feel 12 months from now.

You hold the pen that writes your story over the next year no matter where you are today, or how you are feeling or "who" you are fighting (especially if it's your own thoughts and mindset).

Before you there are two doors.

Behind door No. 1, the chance to lean into life and lay the foundation now for your big dreams later, because the work you do today is the fastest path forward.

Behind door No. 2, the option of giving up and giving in. But, you know in your heart of hearts that door No. 2 is not for you! Not a chance. You will choose to lean in strong and keep going through this COVID merry-go-round. Committed to getting better every day. Not letting negative thoughts and outside influences get in your way. If you do those things, then your future looks very bright, indeed.

Short-term pain brings long-term gain

This is practically a law of nature. If you do the right things today, it may not pay off tomorrow or even next week, but you can be damn sure you'll get rewarded eventually. You cannot fail with the right amount of patience, persistence and perspiration (just remember to apply deodorant).

The effort when no one's watching, when you struggle through a workout you'd rather skip, is the fastest path to "overnight success."

So, let's keep going, my friend. Yes, we must always confront the realities of our current challenges, and sometimes you'll lose the little battles along the way when life kicks your behind.

But with enough patience and persistence, and a belief you are capable of so much more, success is inevitable.

A half-dozen years ago I stood atop the Stratosphere in Las Vegas and jumped... 260 meters straight down. The fall is so far you literally run out of scream, have time to take a breath and then start screaming again.

I still remember that moment where my body transitioned from free fall to suspension just before the ground.

The terrifying fall ended, and my brain registered immense relief that I was no longer at risk of imminent death. It was magical, cathartic, freeing.

Truly like I imagine watching the Winnipeg Jets win a Stanley Cup will be.

But now that I think about it, the entire experience wasn't much different than the roller-coaster ride you must endure to see a weight-loss goal through.

Up one moment, when the scale rewards you with validation.

In a terrifying free fall the next, you end up diving into the pantry for some store-baked oatmeal-chocolate chip cookies (been there).

Sudden triumph followed by frustration and failure. Leading to a roller-coaster of emotions. Then you get to do it all over again.

It's no secret you'll need to endure a few ups and downs on the way to success in your fat-loss journey.

One common theme I've noticed among the successful is they reflect on what they could do better the next time they slip up.

They don't play the blame game. Instead, they get brutally honest. Rather than thinking the problem is outside of themselves and their choices, they reflect, take feedback from their coach or mentor and change things enough to do better next time.

Instead of accepting defeat, ask yourself: 'What could I change to make sure the same scenario doesn't play out exactly the same way?'

So take an honest look at what you're doing if it isn't working.

If you default to blaming programs, hormones or a lack of time, you won't look for solutions. You'll just look to reinforce the reasons why you can't get it done.

Two ways to rationally reflect and adjust your plan: re-frame success and failure.

Don't look at your behaviour-changing attempts as either a success or failure. Instead, see each one as the first of a series of episodes in your journey. Reflect on what worked and what didn't, then tweak things to improve.

Instead of accepting defeat, ask yourself: 'What could I change to make sure the same mistake doesn't happen next time?'

If something doesn't work, first look to adjust the plan. Instead of seeing it as a failure, redesign the plan to make it more manageable to follow.

It's not that you can't lose fat, but the way you're approaching fat loss could be setting you up to fail.

For example, if you keep trying the same low-carb diet only to fall off after a few weeks, maybe it's not worth another attempt.

Likewise, if you struggle with late-night snacking or binge-eating, having bags of chips and chocolate in the house on a Friday night can lead to 5,000-calorie crashes that destroy a week's worth of healthy eating.

You must have systems in place. Doing the wrong thing once can destroy the results of doing the right thing 10 times.

So, instead of thinking about adding a new diet or more exercise, first look at what you can subtract from your daily routines and habits that might be holding you back. Addition through subtraction.

I recommend clients write out a NOT to-do list that summarizes a handful of things that always get in their way on the road to health and fitness. That includes setting up your environment to minimize these common pitfalls from happening.

Whenever I want to accomplish something great it comes down to getting clear on where I want to be a year from now, putting a man-ageable plan in place and getting the accountability and support to see it through.

LIVE LONGER FORMULA?

This is a fat loss book, but I'd be remiss if I didn't dive into one of the reasons we work hard on our health in the first place – so we don't lose it!

I'm dedicating a couple chapters to the current science on longevity, A.K.A not dying prematurely.

No one dies "suddenly" of a heart attack, or has a leg amputated due to diabetes out of the blue — these diseases have been working beneath the surface for decades in many cases. So let's present the case for prevention.

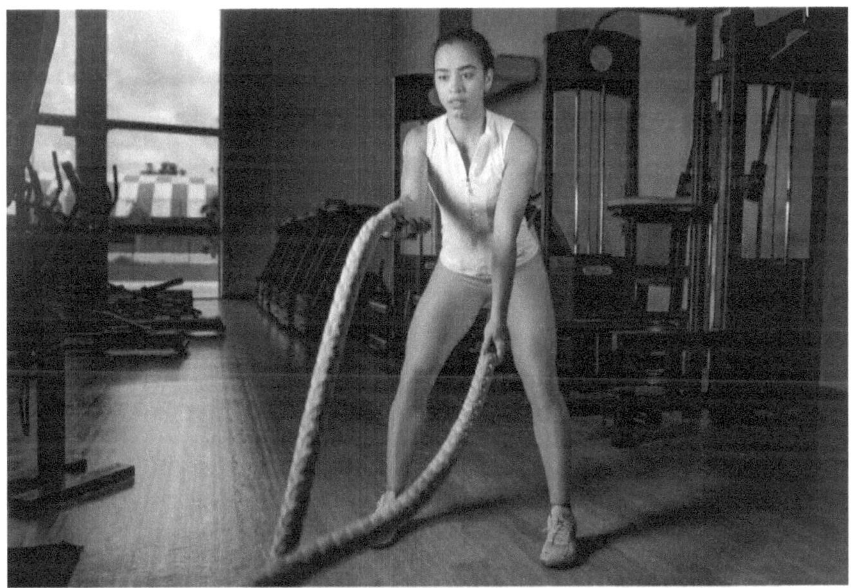

Jonathan Borba / Pexels

You've probably heard of the "Four Horsemen" to avoid in pursuit of living longer: cancer, heart disease, Alzheimer's disease and metabolic disease, such as diabetes.

Insulin resistance is the lead domino for all four aging diseases, according to Attia.

It occurs when cells in your muscles, fat and liver no longer respond well to insulin and can't easily take up glucose from your blood. Visualize a bathtub overflowing with water — fat in this case — from an excess of calories relative to your ability to burn it off or store it in the muscle and liver. This leads to fat storage around your organs (visceral fat), in the liver (fatty liver disease) and around muscle tissue.

"Studies have found that insulin resistance itself is associated with huge increases in one's risk of cancer (up to twelvefold), Alzheimer's disease (fivefold), and death from cardiovascular disease (almost sixfold)."

Most believe diet — and particularly calorie restriction — is the key to longevity, but Attia argues exercise is the more powerful longevity "drug" we have at our disposal.

What can you do in terms of a fitness regimen to increase longevity? Three types of exercise are highlighted in the book: Zone 2 training; VO2 max training; and strength training (with a focus on developing grip strength).

(Disclaimer: Don't get overwhelmed here and aim for perfection. Even going from zero weekly exercise to 90 minutes per week can reduce your risks.)

Zone 2 training

Zone 2 training is any form of cardio (think brisk walk, jogging, stationary bike-riding) done at a moderate pace you can sustain for 30-plus minutes while barely being able to have a conversation.

A Zone 2 workout should feel "kinda sweaty" without major "muscle burn" (excess lactic acid in the muscles).

As you do Zone 2 training, you are training the mitochondria in your muscle cells (the cell's power plants) to use fat as fuel.

VO2 max training

VO2 max training is "embracing the suck" involving exercise that has you go all-out — to the point you can only sustain it so long before needing a recovery period. Think sprinting sports such as hockey or basketball.

The test you may have seen for this occurs in NHL combines, for example, where a player puts an oxygen mask on and goes all-out maximum for four minutes, easy for four minutes, for four rounds. It's rough.

A home-based, safer version to try would be a max-effort sprint at a high resistance on a stationary bike, followed by a recovery period (for example, 30 seconds maximum effort, one- to two-minute recovery pace). Please consult your medical professional before attempting.

The science is clear — if you increase VO2 max to above-average capacity for your age, you reduce your risk of dying prematurely by 50 per cent! Nothing else compares to that.

Strength training

Strength training vastly improves metabolic health because it creates more lean muscle mass that soaks up excess sugar like a sponge.

It literally gives you an extra storage locker for carbs. Yum. More importantly from a longevity perspective, strength is strongly linked with living longer.

A 10-year study of 4,500 subjects over 50 found those with low muscle mass and strength were three times more likely to die early.

Set a strength-training target to lift weights, full body, three times a week for 30 minutes if you're just getting started.

It's insane to think you should stop after the age of 50 — this becomes more important the older you get. You're sore because you're not doing this.

If you're more advanced, you can split up the training sessions by muscle group and take on more sessions per week.

Focus on grip strength (exercises like the farmer's carry — carrying a dumbbell in each of your hands), but nearly every exercise involving moderate to heavy weight will work your grip.

Your goal is to be able to do a farmer's carry for one minute while holding half your body weight in each hand.

One study even claims that grip strength is better at predicting premature death than blood pressure.

The reason could be that a lack of strength indicates accelerated DNA aging, which is linked to disease and disability.

That's the exercise plan on paper. Not easy to execute, but your life may very well depend on making it happen!

Three diet tips for living longer

Now we focus on what science recommends you do in terms of diet to extend quality and length of life.

The good news is you don't have to starve yourself to live longer, like the fasting community claims. Nor do you need to restrict carbs to zero or follow any one diet style.

But there are three eating rules anyone without kidney damage can follow to extend life, according to Attia.

1. Consume an amount of protein indexed in grams to one's weight in pounds to maintain lean muscle.
    Muscle helps you defy the most common challenges of getting older, so a 195-pound person would strive for 195 grams of protein each day. It's best to space out that amount over three to five meals and snacks to optimize muscle retention and digestion.

2. Don't eat heavily (or at all) within three hours of bedtime.
    Eating too near bedtime reduces slumber quality, and sleep is a must as we age. This also includes drinking alcohol, which destroys REM sleep if we consume it too close to bedtime.

3. Stick to an eating plan that keeps average blood sugar in a safe range.
    Get blood work done and check your fasting blood-glucose levels and HbA1c, which is your average blood-glucose (sugar) levels for the last two to three months. Those tests will give your doctor a good read on things.

But you could take it a step further still. The technology now exists for continuous glucose monitoring with real-time feedback. You could start with a simple drugstore glucose monitor and take blood-sugar readings after meals (a good rule of thumb is to see your blood sugar dropping within an hour afterwards and not exceed 8.9 mmol/L)

Keeping your blood sugar in check is key to reducing risk of the Four Horsemen diseases, but how you should eat to achieve this is highly individualized. It's based on one's age, activity levels and muscle mass.

The basics work best here. Eat whole foods, keep calories under control, prepare more meals from scratch, consume protein and produce, control your carb intake (lower if sedentary and higher if really active) and eat to 80 percent fullness.

Don't overthink it — focus on reducing overall calorie intake, getting enough protein and finding the right mix of fats and carbs to support your goals, while not eating to excess.

There are also intangibles that facilitate living longer and healthier beyond diet and exercise that Attia touches on. Prioritizing your sleep and creating a consistent routine promotes better physical and cognitive performance.

Your emotional health is just as vital, so addressing issues like depression or trauma can contribute to your overall well-being. Connecting with other human beings and not isolating yourself also goes a long way.

By focusing on all these areas, you can work toward a fulfilling, active and healthy life, and live as long as humanly possible while thriving along the way.

SARCO-WHAT?

Yes, most forget a secret ingredient to longevity: muscle mass. Sounds basic, but stick with me; science has my back.

What's the big deal about muscle? In a nutshell, muscle mass is like a biological retirement account. Invest early and often, and you're set for a golden age that's truly golden. Skip the muscle-saving, and you might end up like an RRSP you don't invest in — not much help for you in later years.

Before we dive into why muscle is your ticket to the "Forever-Young Club," let's chat about sarcopenia. Sounds like a pasta dish, but it's far less appetizing. It's a skeletal-muscular disorder characterized by a gradual loss of muscle mass, strength and functionality. Signs include slow walking speed, muscle weakness and a hard time with everyday activities such as climbing stairs.

Getting old comes with some baggage, including a higher risk of falls, fractures, hospitalization and, yes, risk of accidental death. Sarcopenia speeds up after the age of 60, with men losing muscle strength at a rate of three to four per cent per year and women at 2.5 to three per cent. But the work you do (or don't do) in your 40s and 50s plays a major role in whether you age gracefully, too.

Many conversations I have go one of two ways when I preach about the importance of muscle. Many women do not want "too much" muscle because they fear they'll get bulky (hard to do without anabolic steroids!). At the same time, aging men who lifted weights when they were younger often lean towards low-impact activities, such as yoga or walking, thinking they're safer and more age-appropriate.

But I'd argue strength-training (and a diet that supports muscle maintenance) is more important than mobility as you get older. If your muscles are more robust, you improve your quality of life.

According to Dr. Gabrielle Lyon, muscle isn't just for looking good and performing well, but those who are stronger have better outcomes fighting off disease.

Why? Lyon says muscle is your amino-acid reservoir, and all your organs and tissues, including brain, liver and kidneys, need a steady flow of amino acids. Therefore, muscle can help sustain you during fasting, injury and illness, giving you a better chance of survival when the going gets tough.

We often blame obesity for diseases like diabetes and cancer, but Lyon argues part of the problem is a lack of muscle mass as well.

The more robust and healthier your muscles, the more carbohydrates and fat your body burns at rest and during exercise.

Plus, muscle is a storage locker for excess glucose, so if you're under-muscled and eating too much, where does that extra glucose (carbohydrates) go? This excess of sugar in the bloodstream is the eventual cause of insulin resistance, which has links to diseases such as diabetes and cancer.

The message is clear: what you do in your 40s and 50s matters, but even if you're in the thick of your 60s, you can still do plenty to reverse sarcopenia and age gracefully.

Flex your way to longevity

You can't control getting older, but you can control how you age. And if you want a shot at becoming the coolest, fittest grandparent on the block, investing in muscle mass is non-negotiable. So, whether you're a fitness newbie or a gym rat, remember: your muscles aren't just for show — they're your ticket to a healthier, more vibrant life.

Ready to age like fine wine? A comprehensive review of 18 random-ized, controlled trials established that increased protein intake com-bined with resistance training is the secret sauce for maintaining muscle strength and mass. Start lifting those weights and filling up on protein. Your future self will thank you.

Starting in your 30s, you lose about three to eight percent of your muscle mass per decade, and more after turning 60. Bone mineral density also starts to decline in midlife, which puts you at risk for frac-tures and osteoporosis. Your VO2 max, the heart and lungs' ability to take in oxygen and convert it into energy during exercise, decreases naturally as well.

First, it's important to figure out what you want your body capable of doing in your 60s, 70s and beyond.

Do you want to be able to squat down and pick up your grandkids? Better squat now. Do you want to be able to travel to Europe without a wheelchair or walker? Better walk plenty of hills now. Do you want to be able to play pickleball or walk around your neighbourhood? Better do those things now.

Strength training is your best defence against bone loss.

Making a few changes to your habits early can slow these declines and prepare you for decades of physical activity.

The problem is the compound effect. Our bodies are quite capable of maintaining homeostasis (fairly stable conditions necessary for sur-vival) when we're younger, but that capability declines over the years. It's one reason we need three days to recover from a late night on the weekend, something we'd easily brush off without issue in our 20s!

But the costs catch up to us in our 40s and 50s if we don't prioritize our health.

What do you prioritize so you can live quality years chasing 100? The key areas to get in check are your body's stability (lump flexibility and mobility here too), strength and cardiorespiratory fitness.

For stability, you'd want a functional-movement screening done. Maintaining balance during standing is a fundamental human skill, and is predictive of falls as we age if it isn't addressed.

If your balance scores are low, start doing balance-boosting exercises like single-leg stands, or workouts like tai chi or pilates. Or if you're less flexible than you desire, take up yoga or devote more time to dynamic stretches. Strength training can absolutely help here, as stretching a muscle under load is very effective for flexibility.

Next up is strength, which is strongly linked with living longer.

A 10-year study of 4,500 subjects over 50 found those with low muscle mass and strength were three times more likely to die early.

It's insane to think you should stop after 40 — this becomes more important the older you get. You're sore because you're not doing this.

One strategy most adopt is to use exercise as a tool to burn as many calories as possible in circuit workouts, boot camps and so on.

The problem with that option is just how ineffective it is. A hard one-hour workout might help you burn 400 calories, easily negated by a latte and doughnut.

And, once the workout is finished, your body tries to conserve calories in other ways to make up the energy deficit. You're wiped out and hungry, moving less and eating more the rest of the day so the net "gain" is even lower. It's a survival mechanism that unfortunately doesn't serve us very well nowadays.

Plus, your body learns to get better at whatever workout you do. The first time you do that mile run you may burn 500-plus calories, but weeks later you're more efficient and burn just half that amount in many cases.

Studies also show weight loss from diet and cardio alone — in the absence of strength training — results in as much as half of the weight loss coming from lean muscle. That means your body burns fewer calories over time, and gets weaker overall. Not a good thing for long-term success.

Another strategy is to get leaner without getting a whole lot lighter. How do we do this? By building muscle! With resistance training you are primarily asking your body to become stronger and, since muscle is a very active and calorie-hungry tissue, your metabolism burns more calories at rest over time.

The best part is the "compound interest" of resistance training doesn't require daily deposits to pay off. For most people who are looking for a fit, healthy body with a speedier metabolism, two to three days a week of 30- to 45-minute resistance-training workouts is more than enough.

If you've been training for a few years, though, look at it in terms of total weekly sets per muscle. You need to find the minimum effective volume your body needs per week to progress. For an intermediate that might be somewhere in the 10-12 sets per muscle group range, and likely more for an advanced trainee, depending on the intensity of your working sets.

Here's one way we'd structure a sample upper-body workout for someone with a few years of training experience who trains three times per week.

1a. Upper push (dumbbell press)

1b. Upper pull (back rows)

2a. Upper push stretch (chest fly)

2b. Upper pull stretch (dumbbell pullover)

3a. Biceps (incline seated dumbbell curls)

3b. Triceps (CG pushups)

4a. Forearms (hammer curls)

4b. Triceps stretch (overhead dumbbell/rope extensions)

5. Anaerobic abs (for example, planks and squats, 30 seconds on, 10 seconds off, for five minutes)

We strategically use "non-competing" muscle groups in super sets to avoid strength drop-off while maximizing time efficiency.

Finally, did you know one in two women and up to one in four men will break a bone in their lifetime due to osteoporosis?

Or that half of all people age 50 and older are at risk of breaking a bone due to poor bone health?

Strength training is your best defence against bone loss. Hopefully that's convinced you to pick up some weights. It'll do you good.

In the end, your goal is to choose activities that minimize time commitment and maximize return on investment. Think short strength workouts, sitting less and short bursts of mobility work to keep you rolling along into your later years fighting back against Father Time.

BRAIN AND BODY CONNECTION

It's hard to have a healthy brain in an unhealthy body. The brain and body are connected through neural pathways made up of neuro-transmitters, hormones and chemicals.

When the body breaks down, brain cells can become damaged. This damage interferes with the ability of brain cells to communicate with each other. When brain cells cannot communicate normally, thinking, behaviour and feelings can be affected.

That's essentially what causes dementia, and in today's chapter we're going to discuss this disease and how to reduce your risk of getting it. Dementia is not a single disease; it's an overall term — like heart dis-ease — that covers a wide range of specific medical conditions, includ-ing the most common, Alzheimer's disease.

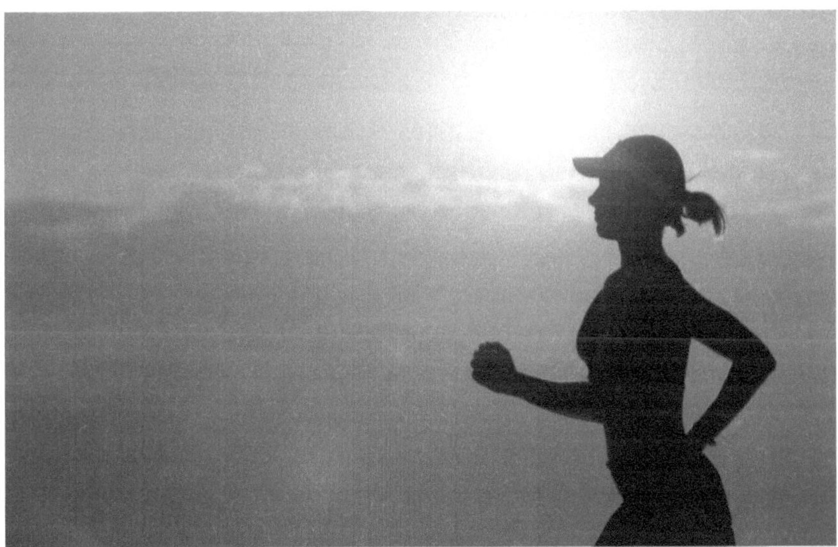

Pixabay / Pexels

Dementia is a general term for loss of memory, language, problem-solving and other thinking abilities that are severe enough to interfere with daily life.

Approximately one out of every 14 people over 65 gets diagnosed with dementia. That is far too many, and, unfortunately, numbers are trending upward. Some experts expect that number to double in the next 20 years.

What causes it? Every month there seems to be a study suggesting another new link to dementia. Last month, new research out of the University of California-San Francisco found a link between popular prescription (and some over-the-counter) sleep medications and the risk of developing dementia.

Another report in the journal *Neurology* back in February found the use of laxatives regularly might increase the risk of dementia as well.

Then there are the usual culprits. A 2018 study found that nearly one-third of early-onset dementia cases were directly linked to alcohol. Other research shows smoking can increase the risk of dementia, especially if you're 65 or older.

Of course, there's a difference between correlation and direct causation, and these reports aren't fully conclusive. Nonetheless, it's concerning that common medications and lifestyle choices so many partake in have strong links to dementia.

So what can you do as an individual to reduce your risk? Well, thankfully we have some answers. A recent study — conducted by the Lancet Commission and shared by Arnold Schwarzenegger in his email newsletter — identified 12 behaviours that can help delay or prevent your chance of dementia by 40 per cent.

Here are the 12 behaviours in no particular order:

- After the age of 40, maintain a systolic blood pressure of 130 mm Hg or less.

- Limit your alcohol intake to a maximum of two to three drinks per week.

- Connect with friends at least three times per week. This can involve phone calls, texts, coffee, meals, Zoom or FaceTime. Do what it takes and make sure you're not socially isolated.

- It may seem obvious, but stop smoking and support others to stop smoking. Secondhand smoke is also associated with dementia.

- Take daily walks.

- Do some sort of resistance exercise (strength training) two to three times per week.

- Avoid obesity. That means having a Body Mass Index (BMI) of less than 30. But, if you have a lot of muscle, BMI isn't always the best measure. In that case, you can use other measurements to assess your health. Men should try to keep their waist size under 38 inches and women under 35 inches.

- Keep your blood pressure under 130/85, and fasting blood sugar under 100 mg/dl. (Of course, consult your physician on any of these numbers.)

- Stop wearing headphones at maximum volume. Hearing loss is associated with the development of dementia. And, if you develop hearing loss, use hearing aids.

Ultimately, the things you know you should be doing tend to highlight this list, and as expected, exercise is chief among them. A 2019 study showed aerobic exercise may slow shrinking in the hippocampus, the part of the brain that controls memory.

Another 2019 study revealed active older adults tend to hold on to cognitive abilities better than those who are less active.

If you have a serious health condition, talk to your doctor before starting a new exercise regimen. And if you haven't exercised in a while, start small — even 15 minutes of daily walking goes a long way. I recently read a story profiling a 98-year-old woman, Betty McKeown, of Elgin, Ill., who walks three miles every day and swears it's what keeps her young.

The best sustainable thing you can do for your health and longevity over the course of your life is to walk every day.

But if you're already getting plenty of steps in, you may want to take it a step further. Scientists recently compared behaviours that impact the brain by assessing the benefits of fasting, light exercise and intense workouts. They measured BDNF (Brain-Derived Neurotrophic Factor), a chemical that supports the health, longevity, size and strength of your brain.

It might surprise some, but fasting had no impact on BDNF in this study. Doing light exercise led to a small increase. But it was hard exercise that made the biggest difference. Just six minutes of intense intervals triggered a five-fold increase in BDNF, compared to the lower-intensity workout.

This adds to the growing science pointing to the fact exercise is "fertilizer" for your mind and body. Not only does movement help protect against degenerative disease, but it might also help make your mind sharper and keep your brain young.

The study suggests you don't need to do two-a-day workouts to get results. The benefits were seen after just six minutes. But, for the biggest boost to brain health, you may want to focus on intensity. That can be done through short spurts of exercise that get your heart rate up, like sprinting on a stationary bike, strength training with heavy weights or circuit workouts.

Consider this one more reason why exercising is worth the effort.

PUTTING IT ALL TOGETHER ("PERFECT MEAL PLAN")

So, you've got this far, why not reward you with an actionable blueprint to take with you!

To reiterate, head to www.mitchcalvert.com/calculator to determine your EXACT custom CAP (Calorie & Protein) target.

But, assuming you've taken that step already, I'm going to give you a template to work with.

Here's one sample meal plan for a 200-pound person looking to lose one to two pounds per week.

Their calorie goal is roughly 2,000 (plus or minus 10% above or below that number is fine) with a protein goal in the range of 170-200g per day. Please read the disclaimer at the front of the book and don't follow this template without first consulting your trusted health care professional.

Breakfast: Balanced Beginnings

- Scrambled Eggs and Toast
- 2 large eggs (100g): 12g protein, 1g carbs, 10g fat
- 2 egg whites: 7g protein, 0g carbs, 0g fat
- 2 slices whole wheat toast (60g): 6g protein, 24g carbs, 2g fat
- 1 medium banana (118g): 1.3g protein, 27g carbs, 0.4g fat

    - Total for meal: 26.3g protein, 52g carbs, 12.4g fat

Mid-Morning Snack: Yogurt Parfait

- Greek Yogurt with Berries and Honey
- 150g Greek yogurt: 15g protein, 6g carbs, 0.3g fat
- 100g mixed berries: 1g protein, 14g carbs, 0.5g fat
- 1 tablespoon honey (21g): 0g protein, 17g carbs, 0g fat

    - Total for snack: 16g protein, 37g carbs, 0.8g fat

Lunch: Chicken Quinoa Salad

- Grilled Chicken Breast with Quinoa and Veggies
- 150g grilled chicken breast: 45g protein, 0g carbs, 3g fat
- 100g cooked quinoa: 4g protein, 21g carbs, 1.8g fat
- Mixed salad greens and veggies (100g): 2g protein, 10g carbs, 0g fat
- Olive oil & lemon juice dressing (1 tablespoon each): 0g protein, 1g carbs, 14g fat

    - Total for meal: 51g protein, 32g carbs, 18.8g fat

Afternoon Snack: Protein Smoothie

- Protein Shake with Fruit
- 1 scoop whey protein vanilla (30g): 24g protein, 3g carbs, 1g fat
- 200ml almond milk: 1g protein, 3g carbs, 2.5g fat
- ½ cup frozen mango (75g): 0.5g protein, 15g carbs, 0.3g fat

    - Total for snack: 25.5g protein, 21g carbs, 3.8g fat

Dinner: Fish and Sweet Potato

- Baked Salmon and Sweet Potato
- 125g cooked salmon: 29g protein, 0g carbs, 7g fat
- 200g baked sweet potato: 4g protein, 41g carbs, 0.3g fat
- Steamed asparagus (100g): 2.2g protein, 4g carbs, 0.2g fat

    - Total for meal: 35.2g protein, 45g carbs, 7.5g fat

Evening Snack: Cottage Cheese Mix

- Cottage Cheese and almond butter
- 150g cottage cheese: 18g protein, 6g carbs, 2.5g fat
- 1 tablespoon almond butter (16g): 3.5g protein, 3g carbs, 9g fat

    - Total for snack: 21.5g protein, 9g carbs, 11.5g fat

Total Daily Intake

- Protein: 175g
- Carbs: 196g
- Fat: 54.8g
- Calories: Approximately 2,000ish (calculated using generic values; specific brands and preparations can vary)

MEAL IDEAS

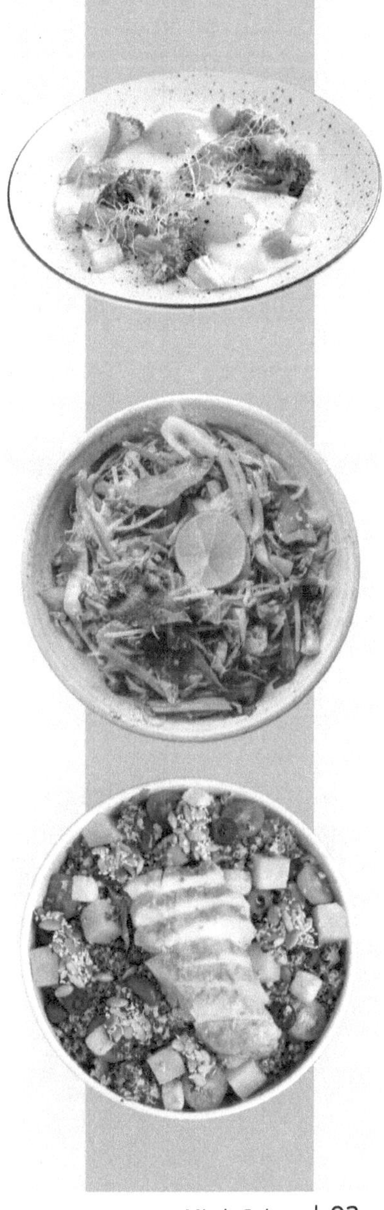

BREAKFAST

Egg scramble with veggies (broccoli, spinach, peppers) + small oatmeal with a little almond butter

Smoothie with almond milk, spinach, ¼ avocado, ½ frozen banana, berries, cinnamon, and protein powder

Turkey sausage with a veggie hash (carrots, sweet potatoes, onions, and peppers) cooked in olive oil

LUNCH

Veggie salad with greens, grilled chicken, and black beans, drizzled with an olive oil-based vinaigrette

Open-faced turkey sandwich with sliced tomatoes and avocado on Ezekiel bread, and a side of fresh-cut veggies

Burrito bowl with lean beef, cauliflower rice, pinto beans, and salsa.

DINNER

Sheet pan salmon + sweet potato + broccoli, all roasted with olive oil

Grilled lean beef burger + rice + green beans

Pan-seared scallops + buckwheat noodles + a veggie stir fry cooked in olive oil

GROCERY LIST

Now that you've got the formula down, here are some foods you can mix-and-match to build new Perfect Plate combinations.

NON-STARCHY VEGGIES

Artichokes
Asparagus
Beets
Brussels sprouts
Broccoli
Cabbage
Carrots
Cauliflower
Celery
Celery
Cucumber
Eggplant
Turnips
Greens
Jicama
Leeks
Mushrooms
Okra
Onions
Peppers
Radishes
Sprouts
Squash (summer)
Swiss chard
Tomato
Zucchini

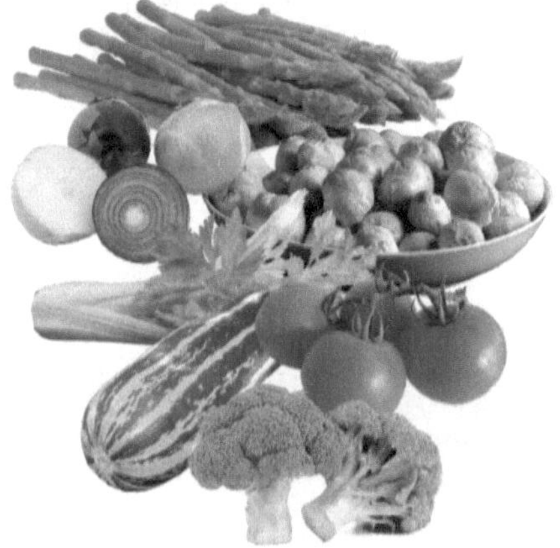

FRUITS

Apple
Apricots
Berries (any kind)
Cantaloupe
Grapefruit
Honeydew
Peaches
Pear
Nectarine
Banana
Cherries
Grapes
Mango
Plums
Oranges
Kiwi
Pineapple
Tangerine

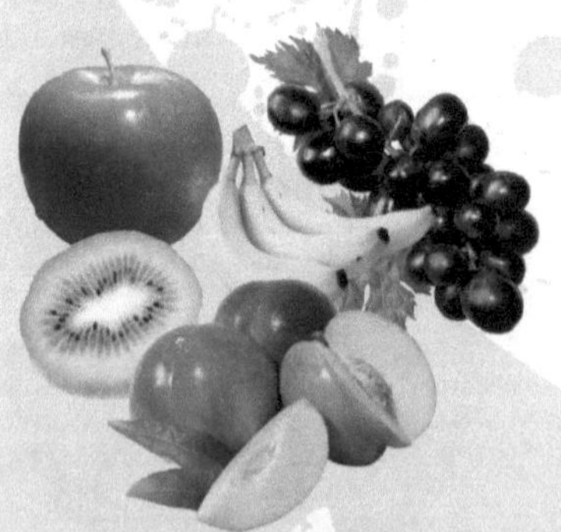

More foods (carbs, protein, and fats) for your mix-and-match combinations.

STARCHY CARBOHYDRATES

Winter squash
Parsnip
Pumpkin
Legumes (Lentils, black beans, etc.)
Whole grain rice
Quinoa
Spaghetti Squash
Sweet Potatoes

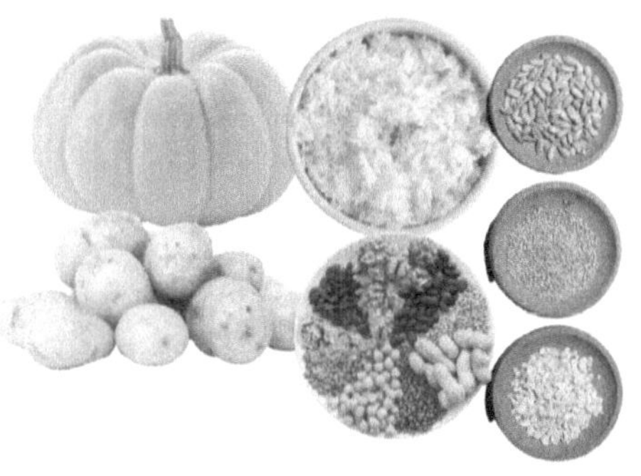

PROTEIN

Turkey
Chicken
Fish
Eggs
Pork
Extra Lean Beef

Seafood
Bison
Tofu
Legumes, like lentils, beans, etc. (for plant-based meals)
Tempeh
Seitan

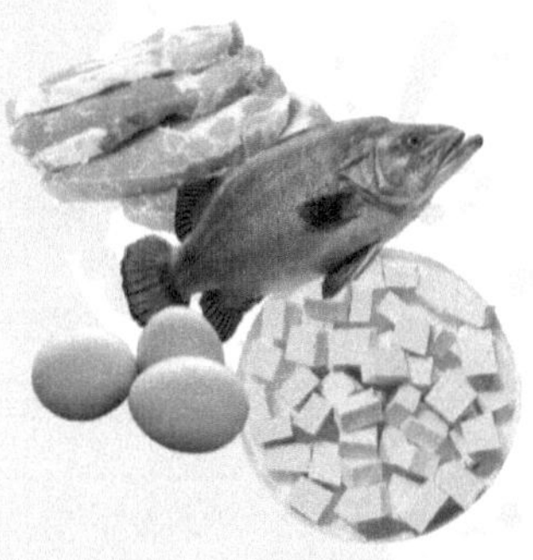

HEALTHY FATS

Extra Virgin Olive Oil
Coconut Oil
Avocado (¼ avocado)

Bacon, 1 slice (limited quantities)
Nuts & nut butters

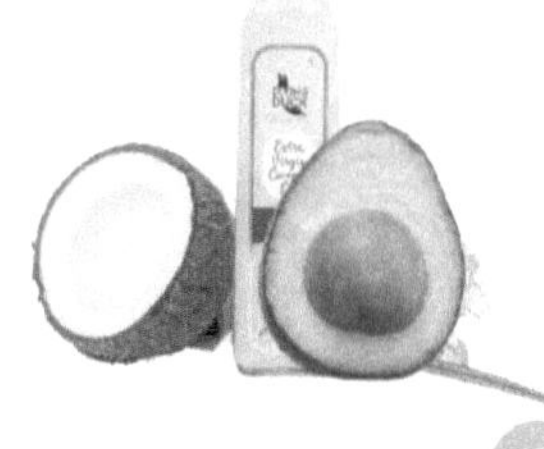

WORKOUT TEMPLATES

Beginner:

Training Template

MON	TUES	WED	THURS	FRI
Lower Strength (Repeated Effort)	Cardiac Output Method	Upper Strength (Repeated Effort)	Cardiac Output Method	Full Body Strength
1. Squat	30-60 minutes of conversational 'cardio' using 3-4 cyclical pieces	1. Upper Press	30-60 minutes of conversational 'cardio' using 3-4 cyclical pieces	1a. Hinge
2. Hinge		2a. Upper Push		1b. Upper Press
3. Single Leg		2b. Upper Pull		2a. Squat or SL
4. Direct Glute		3a. Biceps		2b. Upper Pull
5. Anti Extension		3b. Triceps		3a. Anaerobic Capacity
		4. Anti-rotation		3b. Carry

Intermediate:

Intermediate Client
Training age of 3+ years

MON	TUES	WED	THURS	FRI	SAT
FBT	Tempo Intervals	FBT	Cardiac Output		Walk & Correctives
1a. Squat	20 x 15s hard/45s easy - cyclical	1a. Single Leg	30-40 minutes of Z2 steady-state cyclical.	1a. Hinge	Bird Dogs, Thoracic Rotations, Bear Crawl, ect.
1b. H. Press		1b. V. Press		1b. H. Press	
2a. Hinge		2a. Hinge		2a. Squat	
2b. Upper Pull		2b. Upper Pull		2b. Upper Pull	
3a. Anti-Rotation		3a. Anti-Extension		3a. Anti-lateral flexion	
3b. Direct Biceps		3b. Direct Glutes		3b. Direct Triceps	

*Rest 60-90s between pairings

WHO I HAVE TO THANK

This book wouldn't be possible without all the people that shaped me into the person I am today.

My wife, Brittany, who holds down the fort at home with two kids and two pets while maintaining a full-time job. I don't know how she keeps all the kids' schedules on track, but I know Cal Fit wouldn't be possible without her selfless dedication to everything else.

My parents, who instilled in me an almost delusional belief in myself and what I was capable of. Too often parents dampen their kids' dreams to protect them from failing, but I was lucky to always have their support, no matter how unrealistic my thinking at times.

My early mentors in business, particularly Eric Bach and Craig Ballantyne, who showed me how to not only become a better businessman, but man in general.

My most recent mentor, Vince Del Monte, who helped me break my glass ceiling of income and impact. The best part is the community of other coaches I've connected with over the last three years. Napoleon Hill called this the Mastermind Principle, which he defined as "when people work in perfect harmony for the attainment of a specific purpose." By being around people playing up a level you can "borrow" education, experience, and sometimes even belief.